Lab Values For Nurses

Every Single Lab Value You Must Know To Easily Pass Nursing School & The NCLEX!

2ND Edition

Chase Hassen

Nurse Superhero

© 2017

NurseSuperhero.com

Nclexlabvalues.com

Disclaimer:

Although the author and publisher have made every effort to ensure that the information in this book was correct at press time, the author and publisher do not assume and hereby disclaim any liability to any party for any loss, damage, or disruption caused by errors or omissions, whether such errors or omissions result from negligence, accident, or any other cause.

This book is not intended as a substitute for the medical advice of physicians. The reader should regularly consult a physician in matters relating to his/her health and particularly with respect to any symptoms that may require diagnosis or medical attention.

All rights reserved. No part of this publication may be reproduced, distributed, or transmitted in any form or by any means, including photocopying, recording, or other electronic or mechanical methods, without the prior written permission of the publisher, except in the case of brief quotations embodied in critical reviews and certain other noncommercial uses permitted by copyright law.

NCLEX®, NCLEX®-RN, and NCLEX®-PN are registered trademarks of the National Council of State Boards of Nursing, Inc. They hold no affiliation with this product.

Some images within this book are either royalty-free images, used under license from their respective copyright holders, or images that are in the public domain.

© **Copyright 2017 by Chase Hassen & Nurse Superhero. All rights reserved.**

Introduction to Laboratory Values

This course is intended to be a complete discussion of the laboratory values a nurse must encounter as part of his or her practice. When thinking of lab values, it is tempting to think of hematology, or the study of laboratory values that come from taking a person's blood. In reality, laboratory values can come from many sources, including the urine and the spinal fluid. There are even laboratory values that come from arterial blood rather than venous blood. In brief detail, we will first discuss how laboratory values are obtained from each of these sources and then we will commence with a discussion of the laboratory tests you will encounter on the job, in nursing school, and the NCLEX exam.

There are several chapters in this guide. You will learn about the collection of blood and body fluids for laboratory evaluation, the types of tubes and their colored tops that must be drawn in a certain order at the time of the venipuncture, some common lab test abbreviations, and a wide collection of information on the types of lab tests you will need to know as part of the NCLEX examination.

To learn about my favorite learning strategies to apply to these topics, visit: www.nursesuperhero.com/learning-strategies

We are excited for you to dive in. Good luck!

Table of Contents

Disclaimer: 2

Introduction to Laboratory Values 4

Chapter 1: Obtaining Laboratory Tests 1

Chapter 2: Tubes for Venous Blood 5

Chapter 3: Laboratory Test Abbreviations 11

Chapter 4: Lab Studies You Need to Know 16
    4.01 Basic Metabolic Panel and Electrolytes 16
    4.02 Arterial Blood Gases 37
    4.03 Complete Blood Count or CBC 49
    4.04 Coagulation Profile Testing 78
    4.05 Cholesterol Panel or Lipid Profile 86
    4.06 Antibody Screening 94
    4.07 Iron Panel 108
    4.08 Kidney Function Tests 115
    4.09 Liver Function Testing 117
    4.10 Lumbar Puncture 125
    4.11 Thyroid Function Tests 128
    4.12 Urinalysis Testing 136
    4.13 Stool Analysis 140

Chapter 5: Top 20 NCLEX Lab Values & Bonus Case Studies 144

Chapter 6: Mnemonics for Lab Values 171

Summary 183

Chapter 1: Obtaining Laboratory Tests

Most laboratory tests will come from venous blood but there are other sources as well. Here are some ways that laboratory testing is obtained:

- **Venous Sampling.** This is also called a venipuncture. Blood is taken after prepping an area of an antecubital vein, a vein in the forearm, or a vein in the back of the hand. Most prep solutions are isopropyl alcohol, applied via a cotton ball or a swab. Alternatively, povidone iodine can be used to prep the area. The blood is sampled via a small 22-gauge needle if the vein is small and is drawn up into a syringe before being transferred to the appropriate tubes. If the vein is large, a vacutainer with an 18-gauge or 20-gauge needle is used to access the venous blood and the blood is directly drawn up into the designated tubes. Hemostasis is achieved by direct pressure using a cotton ball and a piece of tape or Band-Aid is applied.

- **Arterial Sampling.** The main reason for arterial sampling is to obtain arterial blood gas sampling. An area over the radial artery is prepped three times with povidone iodine in order to make sure the area is sterile. A special needle and syringe designed for arterial blood sampling is obtained by palpating the radial artery and getting blood directly from the artery. Hemostasis is achieved by applying direct pressure with a cotton ball for at least three to five minutes as bleeding from this site is common. A pressure bandage is applied to maintain hemostasis. If the patient has an arterial line in place, there is no reason to draw from another artery. Simply obtain sterility from the sample site with povidone iodine and draw the arterial blood from the tube. Arterial blood samples should be kept on ice and evaluated as soon as possible for the most accurate test results.

- **Urinalysis and Urine Culture.** Important information is obtained from sampling the patient's urine. Ideally, urine samples are taken after prepping the urethral orifice with an antiseptic solution and then voiding into a sterile cup, which can be used for both the urinalysis and the urine culture. If the patient can't void or if an extremely sterile sample is necessary, the patient is placed supine and the urethral orifice is cleansed with povidone iodine. A sterile catheter is inserted into the urethra and a sterile sample of urine is obtained and transferred to at least one sterile urine container.

- **Spinal Fluid Analysis.** Spinal fluid might need to be obtained for chemistry evaluation, evaluation for red blood cells and white blood cells, culture, and other testing that might be necessary to diagnose diseases like multiple sclerosis. The patient is placed on their side and is asked to curl up into a ball. An area of the low back is prepped three times with povidone iodine to achieve as sterile a field as possible. An open area between L3 and L4 or between L4 and L5 is found by palpation and a needle is inserted into this area. When it is felt that the spinal space is gotten into, a central stylus is removed from the needle and spinal fluid is seen dripping from the needle. Samples of this fluid are obtained and placed into culture medium and tubes for chemistry evaluation. As there isn't very much spinal fluid, small tubes are used to obtain the spinal fluid.

- **Stool Sampling.** Sometimes a stool sample will need to be evaluated for a culture, fat analysis, or for ova and parasites. Stool is collected usually at the time a bowel movement occurs but small amounts of stool can be obtained from a digital rectal examination. The end result should be a sample of stool in a clean, dry, covered container. For sampling of stool for occult blood, there are commercial cards that allow for a smear of stool to be placed on a portion of the card. The stool is then dried and a drop of solution is placed on the specimen that will detect small amounts of heme in the blood. In collecting a large sample, have the patient urinate first and place a plastic catch container in the toilet to catch the stool. When the stool is collected, use a clean spatula to put a walnut-sized sample of stool or about thirty milliliters of liquid stool in the container. Label the container and place it in a plastic bag. Some stool evaluations can't be done on refrigerated stool samples so ask the laboratory if the sample can be refrigerated. Stool cultures are best done on fresh stool as bacteria can multiply in old stool samples, throwing off the culture results.

- **Wound Sampling.** Wounds may need to be evaluated for culturing. Because the goal is to get a culture, the wound shouldn't be prepared with any antiseptic, which can falsely sterilize the wound fluid temporarily. If the wound is open, anything oozing from the wound, particularly if it is opaque and appears purulent, should be sampled with a sterile cotton swab and placed in a plastic tube designed for this purpose. Most of these tubes will have a glass vial in it that contains saline. Break the saline vial and coat the culture sample with the saline. Some labs prefer to do a culture on a swab that doesn't contain saline so ask the lab before breaking the vial. A Gram stain and a bacterial culture can be obtained from this. If the wound isn't closed, a needle and syringe can be used to aspirate some abscess fluid and this can be cultured directly from the syringe or squirted onto a cotton swab that will be evaluated for Gram staining and culture.

- **Obtaining Blood from an IV Port.** Some patients have an IV in place, which might have fluid running into it or might be closed off with a port. Blood can sometimes be obtained from this site if no other phlebotomy site can be obtained. The IV must be discontinued and flushed with normal saline. A port close to the skin must be chosen and cleaned with isopropyl alcohol. An initial syringe and needle are used to draw up any saline and IV fluid until only blood is available at the port site. Remove the syringe and safely discard it. Then use another sterile needle and syringe to collect the blood and put it into the proper tubes. Flush the IV line and restart the IV. IV ports that have no IV line attached but just have a port should be flushed with heparin to maintain the patency of the IV line.

- **Blood Specimen from a Central Venous Catheter (CVP line).** Patients with a central venous catheter have a unique opportunity to have blood drawn from a central venous site without the need for a needle stick. If there is a single lumen catheter, the infusion must be stopped. If there is a multi-lumen catheter, stop all infusions except those containing vasoactive medications. If vasoactive medications are in the central venous catheter, it might not be a good idea to draw blood from the CVP line. Flush the injection port with saline to get rid of whatever was in the central venous line only after scrubbing the port with isopropyl alcohol for thirty seconds. Waste must then be drawn from the port until only blood is obtained in the syringe. This syringe can be guarded. A sterile syringe and needle or a vacutainer needle can be inserted into the port for the withdrawing of blood. Reattach and reopen the central venous lines and flush the line of any remaining blood.

Chapter 2: Tubes for Venous Blood

There are special tubes that are needed for various kinds of venous blood obtained. Blood must be placed into the proper tube type or the sampling of the blood cannot be obtained accurately. A listing of the tubes necessary for various kinds of blood are included in this segment.

For coagulant blood testing, blood is taken in order to take blood from patients with bleeding disorders or who are on blood thinners that prevent blood from clotting. Blood is evaluated outside the body for things chemistries and other tests but need special attention because the blood will not clot. A gold or a red/gray-topped tube that is also referred to as a tiger tube is a tube that contains a clotting activator. It separates the blood from the serum from the blood using the clotting activator. Tubes with a red top also collect serum and separate the blood. These tubes also contain a clotting activator. Orange-topped tubes or gray/yellow-topped tubes are used to test serum from the blood when the answer is urgently required. Thrombin is in the tube, which rapidly causes clot formation.

Anticoagulant tests are those that don't contain a clot activator but instead have a special additive that binds to the calcium ions in the blood so that the proteins leading to blood coagulation are inhibited. Colors of tubes that contain an anticoagulant include light blue tubes, green tubes, gray tubes, dark blue tubes, lavender tubes, and pink tubes. Hematology specimens are obtained from these types of tubes.

One special type of tube that should be noted is the red-topped tube that doesn't contain a clotting activator. It is used to test for drugs in the blood or for antibodies in the blood. Rarer tubes that don't contain clotting factors include light yellow tubes, tan tubes, and white-topped tubes.

Here are some tubes you need to understand:

- **Yellow Top Tube.** This tube isn't used very often in phlebotomy. It contains sodium polyanethol sulfonate used particularly for blood culture sampling. It is also used for human leukocyte antigen or HLA typing or for conducting genetic testing, such as identifying the parent genotype of a child. Blood culture tubes may also be done with blue tubes, purple tubes, and pink tubes. The pink-topped tube contains soybean-casein broth with CO2 that makes an ideal culture medium for both bacterial and fungal blood culturing.

- **Light Blue Tube.** Tubes that contain light blue stoppers are commonly used in phlebotomy. They contain sodium citrate and CTAD, which is a combination of dipyridamole, adenosine, theophylline, and citrate, which prevent blood clotting. The end result is a whole blood sample that can be used for testing of the partial thromboplastin time or aPTT, protime or PT, fibrinogen level, D-dimer test, or a test for fibrin degradation products.

- **Red Top Tube.** Tubes that have red tops are extremely commonly used in phlebotomy. They are used for both immunohematology and serology testing. If the tube is made from glass, it will have no additives but, if the tube is made from plastic, it will have clot additives and will need inversion to mix the blood with the coagulant. Clotting of the blood happens within thirty minutes. The serum obtained from this tube can be used to evaluate the serum for rheumatoid factor, infectious mononucleosis antibodies, syphilis antibodies, rubella titers, streptococcal antibodies, pregnancy hormone testing, haptoglobin testing, C-reactive protein testing, and cold agglutinin evaluations. Blood is also used from this tube for transfusions, where it measures the person's compatibility with donor cells. This can be used for platelet transfusions, cryoprecipitate transfusions, packed red blood cell transfusions, and transfusions of fresh frozen plasma.

- **Green Top Tube.** Green topped-tubes are used commonly in phlebotomy. They are glass tubes coated with ammonium herapin, lithium herapin, and sodium herapin. These block the normal clotting cascade so whole blood or plasma samples can be obtained from the tube. STAT chemistry testing can be done with this sample and some chemistry testing. Tests that can't be done with these tubes include lithium levels, ammonia levels, sodium levels, or blood banking testing. Green-topped tubes that have a yellow ring on the top are also referred to as plasma separator tubes or PSTs. The have a gel inside that separates the plasma from the packed red blood cells and while blood cells when placed in a centrifuge. Many tests can be obtained from this tube as there will be plasma to test.

- **Purple or Lavender Tube.** These are commonly used in phlebotomy and contain EDTA or ethylenediaminetetraacetic acid, which is an additive that will bind to calcium ions so the clotting cascade is blocked. Whole blood testing, such as a RBC count, hematocrit, hemoglobin, and white blood cell/platelet evaluations can be obtained from this type of tube. They can be used successfully for twenty-four hours; however, if a blood smear on a slide is to be obtained, it should be prepared from the tube within three hours from collection. Less commonly tests performed with a purple top tube include body fluid counts, erythrocyte sedimentation rates or ESRs, sickle cell testing, and reticulocyte counts.

- **Gray Top Tube.** These are used very commonly in phlebotomy. The glass tubes contain sodium fluoride and potassium oxide, or just sodium fluoride, or just Na2 EDTA and sodium fluoride. These are generally used for any labs that need glycolytic inhibition of the blood. Red top tubes can be used for similar testing but gray topped-tubes are preferable when the glucose level can't be assessed right away. Tests that can be used with blood from this tube are numerous, including many routine tests like these:

    o Alcohol level
    o Bicarbonate level
    o Serum lactate level
    o Blood glucose level

- Electrolytes
- Cardiac biomarkers
- Lipid levels and lipid panels
- Endocrine marker testing
- Metabolic testing
- Therapeutic drug level monitoring
- Toxicology testing

- **Less Commonly Used Tubes.** There are many different tubes of colors that can be found in a typical phlebotomy tray. Pink top tubes are used for blood banking and can test for blood antibodies, blood type screening, and cross-matching of blood for transfusion. Royal blue top tubes are usually toxicology testing tubes but can be used to evaluate the blood for trace metals and nutritional markers. Any red top tube with a yellow ring on the top is a serum separator tube. The gel can quickly separate the cells from the serum with centrifugation, yielding serum that can be used for a vast variety of blood testing.

Order of Collection in Phlebotomy Testing

Blood taken in hematology testing needs to be done in a specific order in order to avoid contamination of the contents of one tube into another tube that will not be adequately processed because it contains contaminants. One example of this would be attempting to take a purple top sample from a patient before doing a green top tube. The green top tube will be contaminated with additives from the purple tube, leading to a falsely low calcium level and a falsely elevated potassium level.

The correct order in which tubes should be collected includes the following:

1. Blood culture bottles (a yellow top tube can be used instead) The blood culture bottle with a green cap is for aerobic bacterial cultures and the blood culture bottle with an orange top is for anaerobic bacterial cultures.
2. Yellow top tube for sterile blood cultures. The lab may provide the yellow top tube for aerobic cultures or the culture bottles as noted above.
3. Light blue top tube for coagulation studies and whole blood testing (contains 3.2 percent sodium citrate)
4. Red top tube with a clot activator (contains no preservative) This is used for chemistries, serology, and toxicology.
5. Red top tube with a gel separator (this often has a tiger top with gold in the red top or is just a gold top tube that is also called an SST. Both the red top/gold tube with separator and the gold tube with separator are used for chemistries, serology, and toxicology.
6. Royal blue top tube (contains no preservatives) This is used for trace metal testing.
7. Green top tube that contains heparin. This is used for plasma or whole blood determinations.
8. Green/gray top tube that is also called a PST tube containing heparin
9. Lavender top tube (contains EDTA). This is used for whole blood testing.
10. Pink top tube (contains EDTA). This is used for blood bank testing.

11. Tan top tube (contains EDTA). This is used for blood lead levels.
12. Royal blue top tube (contains EDTA). This is used for trace metal testing in whole blood.
13. Gray top tube (contains acid, citrate, dextrose or ACD). Used for blood banking, paternity testing, HLA phenotyping, and DNA testing.
14. Yellow top tube (contains ACD Solution A or B). This is used for flow cytometry and tissue typing assays.

Memory Jogger **For the order of draw:**

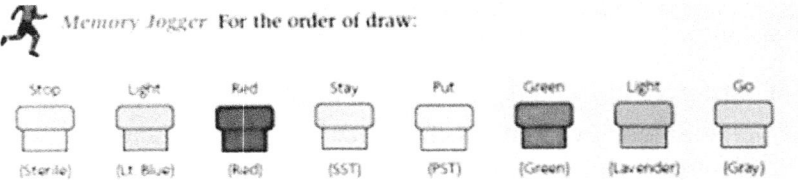

Chapter 3: Laboratory Test Abbreviations

Many blood tests are ordered as an abbreviation rather than written out in longhand formation. The trick is to memorize the abbreviations for these tests so you know which test is being done and which tube to draw the blood from. Here are some of the more commonly-used blood test abbreviations. If you are unsure as to what an abbreviation stands for, always clarify the order with the ordering physician:

- ABG—this stands for arterial blood gas measurement and is done to detect the blood pH level, oxygen level, CO2 level, and bicarbonate level.

- ACE—this stands for angiotensin converting enzyme. ACE inhibitors are often used for blood pressure elevation, kidney protection in diabetes, and heart failure. A level might be drawn of this drug.

- ALP—this stands for alkaline phosphatase and is a test that may be done for liver disease evaluation or for problems in the bones.

- ALT—this stands for alanine aminotransferase, which is a common liver enzyme evaluated when liver diseases like cirrhosis or hepatitis are suspected.

- AST—this stands for aspartate aminotransferase, which is a common liver enzyme. Things like liver failure, cirrhosis, and hepatitis can be evaluated using this test.

- BRCA Gene test—this is a test that should be done when a woman is suspected of having the BRCA gene, which would put her at an increased risk of certain types of breast cancer or ovarian cancer.

- BUN—this is a blood urea nitrogen test, which is a test for dehydration or kidney disease.

- CEA—this stands for carcinoembryonic antigen. The usual test is the CEA-125 or CA-125 test, which is a cancer marker, mostly for female reproductive cancers but other cancers can secrete this tumor marker.

- Ca—This stands for calcium and is a test for various diseases, including parathyroid disease, bone diseases, and some cancers.

- CBC—this stands for a complete blood count. It is a test for all of the blood components, including the red blood cell count, platelet count, and white blood cell counts.

- CMV titer—this stands for a titer for cytomegalovirus. Patients suspected of having cytomegalovirus can use this test to check for the titer of the virus in the blood.

- CPK—this stands for creatinine phosphokinase. It is found in muscle so can be used to check for muscle deterioration; however, a CPK-MB test is an evaluation for cardiac ischemia in a heart attack.

- CRP—this stands for C-reactive protein. It is an often tested when inflammation is suspected or if a heart attack is suspected.

- CSF—this stands for cerebrospinal fluid. This fluid surrounds both the brain and spinal cord and is assessed when brain, spinal cord, or certain diseases need to be evaluated for by doing a lumbar puncture.

- ESR—this stands for erythrocyte sedimentation rate, which is a common test for any kind of inflammation in the body.

- FSH—this stands for follicle stimulating hormone and is a hormone that is checked for when trying to identify fertility issues or when trying to detect the presence of menopause.

- GRF—this stands for glomerular filtration rate, which is a test for kidney failure.

- HBsAg—this stands for hepatitis B surface antigen, which is test for chronic active hepatitis B infections.

- HDL—this stands for high density lipoprotein level and is a test for the "good" cholesterol lipoprotein in the blood.

- HCT—this stands for hematocrit, which is a measurement of the number of red blood cells in a whole blood sample.

- HGB—this stand for hemoglobin, which is a measurement of the protein that carries oxygen in the blood.

- HPV—this stands for human papillomavirus. It isn't usually tested for in the blood but can be tested for in Pap testing or in a biopsy specimen of a suspicious lesion.

- LDL—this stands for low density lipoprotein. It is a test for the "bad" cholesterol lipoprotein and is a measurement often included as part of a lipid profile.

- LFT—this stands for liver function tests and can include several liver enzymes, including the ALT, AST, ALP, and bilirubin.

- Bili—this stands for bilirubin, which is a product of liver metabolism and can be checked for patients with liver dysfunction.

- MRSA—this stands for methicillin-resistant staphylococcus aureus and is something that might be ordered as part of a blood or wound culture.

- PAP—this stands for Papanicolau smear, which is a test done when the cervix is swabbed for human papillomavirus or for evidence of cervical dysplasia.

- PFT—this stands for pulmonary function testing and is a test done by blowing into a tube to assess a person's lung function.

- PPD—this stands for Purified Protein Derivative and is a skin test for tuberculosis.

- PSA—this stands for prostate specific antigen and is a test for benign prostatic hypertrophy or for prostate cancer.

- PT—this stands for prothrombin time and is a test that assesses the effectiveness of warfarin in thinning the blood or for certain blood coagulation disorders.

- PTH—this stands for parathyroid hormone and is a test to evaluate the effectiveness of the parathyroid gland, which secretes this hormone.

- PTT—this stands for partial thromboplastin time and is an assessment of the effectiveness of heparin in thinning the blood or for certain bleeding disorders.

- RF—this stands for rheumatoid factor and is an antibody test that checks for the presence of an antibody that might be present in patients with rheumatoid arthritis.

- RBC—this stands for red blood cell count and is a test for the number of red blood cells in the bloodstream in whole blood collections.

- FANA—this stands for fluorescent antinuclear antibody, which is a test for systemic lupus erythematosus or for several different autoimmune diseases.

- TIBC-this stands for total iron binding capacity and is a test for the amount of protein available in the blood that can bind iron.

- TORCH—this stands for a collection of infectious diseases that are often tested on pregnant women because the infections tested for are teratogenic and dangerous to pregnant women. TORCH may also be known as TORCHS. The acronym stands for toxoplasmosis, "other", rubella cytomegalovirus, herpes simplex, HIV, and syphilis.

- TSH—this stands for thyroid stimulating hormone and is the hormone released by the pituitary gland that stimulates the thyroid gland to release its hormones.

- T4—this stands for thyroxine and is one of the two hormones released by the thyroid gland under the influence of TSH secreted by the pituitary gland.

- T3—this stands for triiodothyronine. It is one of the two hormones secreted by the pituitary gland under the influence of TSH secreted by the pituitary gland.

- LH—this stands for luteinizing hormone, which is a reproductive hormone usually assessed in women to diagnose the time they are ovulating.

- UA—this stands for urinalysis and is the chemistry and microscopic evaluation done on the urine to assess for various metabolic problems and for microscopic evidence of a bladder or kidney infection.

- UC—this stands for urine culture. It is collected under sterile conditions in order to assess the urine for the actual bacterium or bacteria responsible for a bladder or kidney infection.

- WBC—this stands for white blood cell count, which is a measurement of the number of white blood cells in a whole blood sample.

Chapter 4: Lab Studies You Need to Know

The following is an extensive breakdown of all the laboratory tests you'll need to know about in the nursing school as well as the NCLEX examination. Some tests are done as a panel, while other tests are done as individual tests. After studying this part of the guide, you will know what common tests are done and will understand why they might be done and the values you need to look for.

4.01 Basic Metabolic Panel and Electrolytes

The panel of lab values consists of:

- Sodium
- Potassium
- Chloride
- Magnesium
- Phosphorus
- Calcium
- Glucose
- Creatinine
- Blood Urea Nitrogen
- Albumin

Sodium

Abbreviation: Na+

How Is It Measured: Venous blood is taken from a red topped tube, a red/gold tube or a gold tube that has been centrifuged to separate the blood components from the serum.

Description: This test is part of a basic metabolic panel or an electrolyte panel. It is tested with other electrolytes electronically, such as the potassium, phosphorus, chloride, and magnesium levels.

Indications: It is drawn for routine health studies, evaluation for dehydration, evaluation for electrolyte imbalances, weakness, confusion, lethargy, muscle twitching, agitation, or general monitoring of hypertension, kidney disease, heart failure, and liver disease.

Normal Range: Most adults have a normal range of 135-145 mEq/l or mmol/L, while adults greater than 90 years of age have a normal range of 132-146 mEq/L or mmol/L.

Critical Range: Low critical limit for sodium is 120 mEq/L. High critical limit for sodium is 160 mEq/L.

Increased Value May Indicate: Elevated sodium levels or hypernatremia can mean excess water loss in dehydration from any cause such as not drinking enough or diarrheal losses of water. Rarely, a high salt intake can lead to hypernatremia. Patients with diabetes insipidus and Cushing syndrome may have hypernatremia. Rarely, certain antibiotics, steroid use, laxative abuse, birth control pills, and certain cough medications can increase the serum sodium level.

Decreased Value May Indicate: Low sodium levels in the serum is known as hyponatremia. It can be caused by sodium loss in the stool during diarrhea, sodium losses in vomiting, diuretic use, kidney disease, Addison's disease, low aldosterone levels, excessive water intake, and excessive sweating. Any disease that causes SIADH (syndrome of inappropriate ADH) can result in hyponatremia and an excessive reuptake of water by the kidneys. Rarely, low sodium concentrations in IV solutions, low dietary sodium intake, tricyclic antidepressant use, heparin use, ACE inhibitor use, and carbamazepine use can result in low sodium levels.

Factors, Risks, or Other Information: Measurement of the sodium levels in the urine can help diagnose elevated or low sodium levels. Addison's disease and diuretic use can lead to high losses of sodium in the urine, while conditions like congestive heart failure, dehydration, nephrotic syndrome, or liver impairment can lead to low urine sodium levels.

Potassium

Abbreviation: K+

How Is It Measured: This is measured using venous blood and obtaining serum from a red top tube or a red/gold tube with a gel separator that separates the blood components from serum.

Description: This test is done as part of a metabolic panel or electrolyte panel along with sodium, chloride, magnesium, and phosphorus. It is measured electronically along with the other electrolytes and is rarely ordered alone as it is best interpreted as part of a panel.

Indications: The potassium level can be drawn as part of a wellness panel. It is also tested as part of an evaluation for kidney disease, the side effects of using diuretics, evaluation of cardiac arrhythmias, hypertension monitoring, dialysis monitoring, management of diabetic ketoacidosis, and monitoring of patients on intravenous fluids.

Normal Range: The normal range for potassium is 3.5-5.1 mEq/L or mmol/L.

Critical Range: Critically low potassium levels are less than 2.9 mEq/L and critically high levels of potassium are greater than 6.1 mEq/L.

Increased Value May Indicate: High levels of potassium are referred to as hyperkalemia. It can be elevated in patients with Addison's disease, kidney disease, severe tissue injury, sepsis, diabetic conditions, dehydration, excessive potassium intake, or having too much potassium in an intravenous solution. Rarely, some drugs can cause hyperkalemia, such as beta blockers, ACE inhibitors, NSAID medications, and potassium-sparing diuretics (such as spironolactone, amiloride, or triamterene).

Decreased Value May Indicate: Low levels of potassium are referred to as hypokalemia. Hypokalemia can be seen with GI losses in vomiting and diarrhea, hyperaldosteronism (Conn syndrome), insulin intake, potassium-losing diuretic therapy, and acetaminophen overdoses. Rarely, low potassium levels can be seen in corticosteroid use, certain antibiotic use, amphotericin B use, beta-agonist use, and alpha-antagonist use.

Factors, Risks, or Other Information: There ar no risks to having a potassium level drawn. The level is best interpreted along with urine potassium levels. Low levels of potassium in the urine may be seen in the taking of certain drugs like lithium, beta blockers, and NSAIDs. Patients with hypoaldosteronism will have low urine potassium levels. False elevations of the potassium level can be spurious because of the processing of the sample. Delays in getting the level tested or excessive manipulation of the blood sample may cause leakage of potassium from the red blood cells, leading to a falsely elevated potassium level. If the level doesn't match the symptoms, the test needs to be repeated.

•

Chloride

Abbreviation: Cl-

How Is It Measured: Chloride levels are rarely measured as an isolated test but are part of an electrolyte or basic metabolic panel. Venous blood is collected from a red top tube, a red/gold top tube, or a gold top tube. Serum is separated from the whole blood components by centrifugation and the serum level of chloride is measured electronically.

Description: A serum chloride level is drawn as part of an electrolyte panel and the chloride level alone is not diagnostic of anything in particular. Sodium and chloride levels tend to rise and fall together so the indications for a chloride test are basically the same as for a sodium test.

Indications: This test is ordered whenever a patient exhibits evidence of prolonged vomiting or diarrhea. Respiratory distress and weakness can be signs of an electrolyte abnormality involving the chloride level. The chloride level can be abnormal in acid-base disorders, necessitating further testing, such as an arterial blood gas to see if there is an acid-base imbalance.

Normal Range: In most adults, the normal range for chloride is between 98 and 107 mEq/L or mmol/L. In adults over the age of 90, the upper limit for chloride can be as high as 111 mEq/L.

Critical Range: The lower critical value for chloride is 76 mEq/L and the upper critical value for chloride is 125 mE1/L.

Increased Value May Indicate: Elevated levels of chloride are called hyperchloremia, which is most commonly seen in dehydration. Diseases causing elevated sodium levels, such as kidney problems and Cushing disease, will have elevated chloride levels. Chloride is responsive to the acid-base levels in the body so patients who hyperventilate and have respiratory alkalosis will have high chloride levels from a respiratory loss of base in the body.

Decreased Value May Indicate: Low levels of chloride are known as hyperchloremia. Any disease causing low sodium levels will also affect the chloride level. Low chloride levels can also be seen in prolonged vomiting, prolonged gastric suctioning, congestive heart failure, Addison's disease, and certain lung diseases that cause a respiratory acidosis. Patients with metabolic alkalosis from any cause will have low chloride levels.

Factors, Risks, or Other Information: There is no risk to having a chloride level drawn. Certain drugs will alter the chloride level as can over-consumption of baking soda or antacids. The urine chloride level can be measured as a way of interpreting the hypochloremia, with low urine chloride levels seen in CHF, Conn syndrome, Cushing disease, malabsorption, and chronic diarrhea.

Magnesium

Abbreviation: Mg+ or Mag

How Is It Measured: The magnesium level is drawn as part of the basic metabolic and electrolyte panel. The blood is obtained from a red top tube, a red/gold top tube or a gold top tube and the serum is separated from the blood by centrifugation. A sample of serum is tested electronically for all of the electrolytes, including the magnesium level.

Description: This is a serum test that is mainly checked in cases of gastrointestinal disorders, kidney disorders, and uncontrolled diabetes as a way of monitoring these diseases.

Indications: This is a test that is ordered in patients who have muscle wasting disorders, muscle cramping or twitching, cardiac arrhythmias, seizures, confusion, or known hypocalcemia and hypokalemia. Alcoholics with malnutrition may need a magnesium level drawn. Patients with uncontrolled diabetes, kidney disease, or malabsorption syndromes may need a magnesium level drawn.

Normal Range: The normal range is 1.7-2.2 mg/dL

Critical Range: The low critical level for magnesium is less than 1.1 mg/dL, while the high critical level for magnesium is greater than 4.8 mg/dL.

Increased Value May Indicate: Elevated levels of magnesium or hypermagnesemia is rare but it can be seen in patients who take in too much magnesium, hypoparathyroidism, kidney failure, Addison's disease, early diabetic ketoacidosis, dehydration, or the taking of laxatives and antacids that are high in magnesium.

Decreased Value May Indicate: Decreased levels of magnesium is known as hypomagnesemia. It can be seen in patients who are malnourished or alcoholic because of low magnesium intake. Uncontrolled diabetics and patients with malabsorption from Crohn's disease will have low magnesium levels. Hypoparathyroidism, long-term diarrheal illnesses, long-term diuretic use, recent surgery, preeclampsia, eclampsia, and severe burns (which ooze magnesium from burn fluid).

Factors, Risks, or Other Information: There are no risks to having a magnesium level drawn. It is usually best interpreted along with the other electrolyte levels. The potassium level and the magnesium level tend to be low together and physiological hypomagnesemia is seen in the latter half of pregnancy. Remember that the magnesium level does not reflect total body magnesium levels. Magnesium is leached from bone to keep the blood level normal so there can be deficiency states with low bone levels of magnesium and normal serum magnesium levels on blood testing.

Phosphorus

Abbreviation: P or PO4-

How Is It Measured: This test is drawn from venous blood and comes from a red top tube, a red/gold top tube, or a gold top tube after centrifugation to separate the serum from the blood components. It is often drawn as part of a metabolic or electrolyte panel and is determined electronically.

Description: Phosphorus is an electrolyte that is often drawn along with a blood calcium level, the parathyroid hormone level, and the vitamin D level as phosphorus levels are, in part, determined by the parathyroid gland.

Indications: A phosphorus level can be done as part of a screening metabolic panel or electrolyte panel. Mild changes in phosphorus levels are asymptomatic but as phosphorus levels are closely linked to calcium levels, any indication for low or high calcium levels, such as tiredness, cramping, bone pain, or muscle weakness might be an indication for phosphorus testing. Acid-base disorders can affect the phosphorus level so it might be drawn when there is an acid-base abnormality found. The calcium and phosphorus levels are usually drawn and interpreted together.

Normal Range: A normal level of phosphorus for an adult between the ages of 18-60 is 2.7-4.5 mg/dL. Phosphorus levels tend to be higher in children.

Critical Range: A critically low level of phosphorus is 1.2 mg/dL, while a critically high level of phosphorus is 8.8 mg/dL.

Increased Value May Indicate: Elevated levels of phosphorus or hyperphosphatemia can be seen in hypoparathyroidism, liver disorders, kidney failure, early diabetic ketoacidosis, and elevated consumption of phosphate.

Decreased Value May Indicate: A low level of phosphorus is also known as hypophosphatemia. It generally is inversely proportional to the calcium level so it is seen in hypercalcemia secondary to hyperparathyroidism, diuretic abuse, alcoholism with secondary malnutrition, late diabetic ketoacidosis, low potassium levels, severe burns, hypothyroid states, vitamin D deficiency with rickets, and chronic abuse of certain antacids.

Factors, Risks, or Other Information: There are no risks to having the phosphorus level drawn. It should be noted that hyperphosphatemia can cause organ damage from deposits of calcium phosphate in organ tissues. Osteoporosis can be a complication of high phosphate levels. Children will have physiologically-high phosphorus levels because of active bone growth. Overconsumption of phosphorus can happen rarely if individuals consume a great deal of phosphate-containing soft drinks.

Calcium

Abbreviation: Ca+

How Is It Measured: Calcium is drawn from venous blood and from blood taken from a red top tube, a red/gold top tube, or a gold top tube. The serum is separated from the blood cells through centrifugation and the serum calcium is measured electronically, often with other electrolytes.

Description: Calcium is one of several electrolytes measured in a metabolic panel or an electrolyte panel. It is often tested as a way of monitoring diseases of the teeth, kidneys, nervous system, heart, and bones. It is often tested in patients suspected of having hyperthyroidism, a disorder of the parathyroid glands, or any type of malabsorption syndrome.

Indications: Calcium levels can be drawn as part of normal health screening but can be used to measure the status of the parathyroid gland. Urine calcium levels are important to determine along with the serum total calcium level because it can identify whether or not large amounts of calcium are being excreted in the kidneys. The absolute value of the calcium level is less important than the comparison of the calcium level with the parathyroid hormone level, magnesium level, vitamin D level, and phosphorus level. Other indications for testing the calcium level include the evaluation of kidney stones, bone disorders, and symptoms of high or low calcium levels. The main symptoms of hypocalcemia include paresthesias, muscle cramps, and abdominal cramps, while the main symptoms of hypercalcemia include anorexia, thirstiness, increased urination, tiredness, muscle weakness, constipation, stomach pains, nausea, and vomiting. Certain cancers will cause elevated calcium levels so monitoring of the level needs to be done, especially with cancers of the kidneys, lung, and breast.

Normal Range: The normal range for the total calcium level in adults is 8.6-10.2 mg/dL.

Critical Range: A critically low calcium level in adults is less than 6.0 mg/dL, while a critically high level of calcium is greater than 13.0 mf/dL.

Increased Value May Indicate: There are two main causes of hypercalcemia. The main cause is hyperparathyroidism, which usually stems from a benign adenoma of the parathyroid gland. As mentioned, cancers can result in hypercalcemia, especially when they metastasize to bone, causing a leaching of calcium from the bone into the blood. Other cancers will secrete substances that act like parathyroid hormone. Rarely, high calcium levels can be seen in tuberculosis, sarcoidosis, hyperthyroidism, high vitamin D consumption, immobilization, HIV disease, overuse of thiazide diuretics, and in kidney transplant cases.

Decreased Value May Indicate: Most low calcium levels are spurious and are the result of low albumin levels in patients with malnutrition or liver disease. Alcoholics often have low calcium levels. Keep in mind that this is the total calcium level and doesn't reflect the ionized calcium level. Other disorders that can lead to low calcium levels are hypoparathyroidism, low calcium intake, low vitamin D levels, high phosphorus levels, low magnesium levels, kidney failure, and pancreatitis.

Factors, Risks, or Other Information: There are no risks to having a calcium level drawn. High levels of calcium in the blood can lead to kidney stone formation. The total calcium level is closely associated with the ionized calcium level but patients receiving IV fluids, those having a blood transfusion, patients with low albumin levels, and patients having major surgery may need an ionized calcium level instead of a total calcium level. Preterm infants are at a high risk for hypocalcemia and need continual monitoring for this.

Glucose

Abbreviation: Gluc or FBS, which stands for fasting blood sugar

How Is It Measured: The blood glucose level can be checked in many ways. A whole blood sample can be taken from a finger prick and measured separately with a glucose meter on a fasting or non-fasting basis. A yellow top tube can also be drawn and glucose measurements of the blood can be determined. Glucose is often a part of a metabolic panel drawn on a fasting patient.

Description: The glucose level can be high or low. Most testing for glucose involves testing for prediabetes or diabetes and is done on a fasting basis. In some cases, glucose tolerance testing can be done, in which a patient drinks a 100-gram load of glucose in solution and the glucose levels are drawn before drinking the glucose solution and at hourly intervals after drinking the solution.

Indications: There are many reasons to check a blood glucose level as patients can have signs and symptoms of hyperglycemia or hypoglycemia. A fasting blood glucose level can be a screening test for diabetes and prediabetes, while a one-hour glucose tolerance test is evaluated as a screening test for gestational diabetes. Patients with diabetes will monitor their blood sugar levels as they relate to meals and the taking of insulin. The blood glucose level must be very high or very low to be symptomatic, so most fasting and non-fasting blood glucose testing is done to screen people for glucose abnormalities who are otherwise asymptomatic.

Normal Range: A normal fasting blood glucose level is between 70 to 99 mg/dL.

Critical Range: A critically low blood glucose value is less than 51mg/dL in adults, while a critically high blood glucose level is greater than 499 mg/dL.

Increased Value May Indicate: Elevated blood glucose levels are seen in prediabetes and diabetes. There are also diseases that can result in high blood glucose levels. These include Cushing syndrome (with elevated cortisol levels), chronic kidney failure, acute cerebrovascular accident, acute myocardial infarction, trauma, pancreatitis, acromegaly, pancreatic cancer, and hyperthyroidism.

Decreased Value May Indicate: Low levels of glucose or hypoglycemia can cause symptoms, such as anxiety, tremor, hunger, palpitations, and sweating, with severe hypoglycemia affecting the central nervous system, resulting in mental status changes, coma, and death. Diseases that may result in hypoglycemia include low pituitary function, severe liver failure, adrenal insufficiency, excessive alcohol consumption, severe systemic infections, starvation, insulinomas, excessive insulin use, heart failure, and chronic kidney disease.

Factors, Risks, or Other Information: Whether the blood glucose level is drawn from a venipuncture or a finger stick, there is no risk to having this done. It should be known that temporary elevations of blood glucose levels can be seen in surgical situations, major trauma, extreme stress, stroke, or heart disease. Because cortisol levels increase blood sugar, patients taking glucocorticoids will have elevated glucose levels. Other drugs that can raise the glucose level include salicylates, phenytoin, lithium, estrogens, epinephrine, diuretics, and tricyclic antidepressants. Anabolic steroids and acetaminophen can lower glucose levels.

Creatinine

Abbreviation: Creat

How Is It Measured: The creatinine test is a serum test drawn from venous blood. Serum from a red top tube, a red/gold top tube, or a gold top tube can be collected after centrifuging whole venous blood. A serum creatinine level is often done as part of a basic metabolic panel or along with a BUN test as a measurement of kidney function.

Description: The serum creatinine level is highly correlated with an individual's kidney function so it is drawn in order to screen patients with suspected kidney disease or as part of a normal health panel in order to assess the patient's renal function.

Indications: The main indication for doing a serum creatinine level is to evaluate a patient for underlying kidney disease. Diabetics and patients with hypertension carry a risk for kidney disease so a creatinine should be evaluated in these patients. A creatinine level may be drawn prior to surgery or prior to receiving contrast dye to make sure the patient has normal kidney function. The creatinine can be drawn as part of a calculation of the glomerular filtration rate, which is a measure of kidney failure. Clinical indications that suggest renal dysfunction include tiredness, peripheral edema, abnormally-appearing urine, oliguria, poor appetite, flank pain, or hypertension.

Normal Range: The normal range for serum calcium levels is between 0.9 mg/dL and 1.3 mg/dL in adult males and between 0.6 mg/dL and 1.1 mg/dL in adult females.

Critical Range: A critically low creatinine level does not exist as there is no pathology associated with a low creatinine level. A critically high creatinine level is anything greater than 7.3 mg/dL.

Increased Value May Indicate: High creatinine levels usually mean the patient has kidney disease or an illness that affects the function of the kidneys. Acute or chronic kidney damage can cause an elevated creatinine level; autoimmune diseases can affect the kidneys; kidney infections can raise creatinine levels; urinary obstruction can damage the kidneys; any disease that causes low blood flow to the kidneys will result in kidney dysfunction and an elevated creatinine level.

Decreased Value May Indicate: The serum creatinine level is rarely low but is primarily seen in people who have markedly reduced muscle mass. A low creatinine level is not a clinically significant disorder.

Factors, Risks, or Other Information: There can be temporary elevations of the creatinine level unrelated to kidney function but are secondary to muscle injury. Pregnant women have low creatinine levels and certain drugs may temporarily raise the creatinine level.

Blood Urea Nitrogen

Abbreviation: BUN

How Is It Measured: The BUN level is a serum test that is drawn from a venipuncture and is used from blood placed in a red top tube, a red/gold top tube, or a gold top tube from which serum is collected after centrifuging whole blood to separate the serum from the blood products. The BUN is then electronically determined.

Description: The serum BUN test is usually drawn and interpreted along with the serum creatinine test and is a measure of the kidney's overall functioning. Serum BUN levels will be elevated anytime there is an imbalance between the production of urea and the excretion of urea by the kidneys.

Indications: The main indication for doing a BUN test is similar to the reasons for ordering a serum creatinine test. This test will be elevated in acute and chronic kidney failure so it is a good test for monitoring the level of the kidney function. A BUN level may be drawn for signs and symptoms of kidney dysfunction, such as low energy levels, poor appetite, oliguria, flank pain, peripheral edema, or high blood pressure.

Normal Range: The normal range for the serum BUN level is 6-20 mg/dL.

Critical Range: There is no lower limit to a BUN level and no critically low level definable. The upper critical level for the serum BUN level is greater than 104 mg/dL.

Increased Value May Indicate: An elevated serum BUN level almost always means the patient has either acute or chronic kidney disease or kidney failure. Low blood flow to the kidneys, as can be seen in congestive heart failure, heart attack, severe burns, dehydration, stress, or shock, can cause elevations in the serum BUN level. The kidneys can be normal with elevations of the BUN level when protein is excessively broken down as in GI bleeding, muscle catabolism, or increased dietary protein.

Decreased Value May Indicate: There is rarely any need to be concerned about a low BUN level. It can be seen in severe liver dysfunction, malnutrition, and overhydration. Even if one kidney is completely dysfunctional, a second normal kidney can keep the BUN in the normal range.

Factors, Risks, or Other Information: The BUN level isn't as good as the creatinine level in determining kidney function because the level can be elevated with high protein intake and can be low with low protein intake. Pregnancy can artificially raise or lower the serum BUN level.

Albumin

Abbreviation: Alb

How Is It Measured: The albumin test is a serum test derived from a venipuncture in which blood from a red top tube, a red/gold top tube, or a gold top tube is centrifuged to separate the serum from the whole blood products. The serum is collected and the albumin level is obtained electronically.

Description: A serum albumin level is normally a part of a comprehensive metabolic panel used to assess the overall health of normal individuals. It can be low in a variety of diseases so it can be used to monitor treatment status in low albumin diseases. Albumin is the most prevalent blood protein and is necessary for keeping fluid from leaking out of the blood vessels and is responsible for many functions, such as being a carrier protein for drugs, hormones, and some electrolytes. It can be a good measure of an individual's nutritional state.

Indications: The biggest indication for a serum albumin level is for routine health screening. It can be used to evaluate patients with evidence of liver dysfunction, such as jaundice, weakness, dark urine, abdominal swelling, poor appetite, itching, and weight loss. Patients suspected of having nephrotic syndrome with peripheral edema, oliguria, flank pain, and hypertension may have a serum albumin test to evaluate their kidney function. Nutritional status can be evaluated with a serum albumin level.

Normal Range: The normal range for a serum albumin level is 3.5 to 5.0 g/dL in a normal adult.

Critical Range: There are no critical range values established for the serum albumin level.

Increased Value May Indicate: Elevated serum albumin levels are uncommon but can be seen in patients who are dehydrated.

Decreased Value May Indicate: Low serum albumin levels may be seen with plasma volume expansion, liver disease, burns, surgery, infection, congestive heart failure, carcinoid syndrome, hypothyroidism, diabetes, cancer, and certain chronic diseases.

Factors, Risks, or Other Information: There is no risk or danger to having a serum albumin test. It should be noted that patients on intravenous fluids will have inaccurate determinations of their serum albumin level. Drugs, such as insulin, growth hormone, androgens, and anabolic steroids will cause an increased serum albumin determination.

4.02 Arterial Blood Gases

The panel of lab values consists of:

- Base Excess
- Bicarbonate
- Acidity (pH)
- Oxygen Saturation
- Partial Pressure of Carbon Dioxide
- Partial Pressure of Oxygen

Base Excess

Abbreviation: BE

How Is It Measured: The base excess is a calculated value taken from levels ordered in an arterial blood gas assessment. Arterial blood gases are obtained from taking blood from either the radial artery or the femoral artery into a heparinized syringe. All visible gas bubbles are removed from the syringe and the sample is taken on ice to be measured in an arterial blood gas machine.

Description: The base excess level is primarily used for the metabolic assessment of patients with acid-base disorders and is the part of the arterial blood gas test that determines whether the patient has metabolic acidosis or metabolic alkalosis. It is a measurement of the non-respiratory aspect of the pH change in the blood and is calculated based on the HCO_3^- level and the blood pH. The base excess is technically defined as the number of hydrogen ions that would be necessary to return the pH of the blood to a normal value as long as the pCO2 was also normalized.

Indications: The base excess is part of an overall investigation of whether or not a patient has an acid-base disorder. Acid-base disorders can have respiratory components and metabolic components. The base excess measures the metabolic component of a person's pH dysfunction as measured by an arterial blood gas assessment.

Normal Range: The normal range for the base excess is from -3 to +3 mmol/L.

Critical Range: There is no critical range defined for the base excess measurement.

Increased Value May Indicate: As mentioned, the base excess is a calculated level. A base excess higher than +3 mmol/dL is indicative of metabolic alkalosis and suggests a metabolic cause of the pH imbalance.

Decreased Value May Indicate: When the base excess is calculated and is found to be less than -3 mmol/L, the patient is likely to have metabolic acidosis and a workup for this should commence based on this reduced value.

Factors, Risks, or Other Information: Arterial blood gas measurements are generally taken from very sick individuals with both respiratory and metabolic problems contributing to pH abnormalities in the blood. The test is painful and carries a risk of hematoma formation if hemostasis is not maintained for several minutes after taking the blood or if the patient has an underlying bleeding disorder.

Bicarbonate

Abbreviation: HCO3-

How Is It Measured: The bicarbonate level in arterial blood is obtained along with other arterial blood parameters in an arterial blood gas assessment. Blood is taken from the radial or femoral artery into a heparinized syringe that is placed on ice after removing all air bubbles from the sample. The bicarbonate level is then determined by the blood gas analyzer.

Description: The bicarbonate ion is an important aspect of the blood gas analysis. Levels of the bicarbonate in the arterial blood can tell if an individual has metabolic alkalosis or metabolic acidosis. The bicarbonate level alone is insufficient to determine the patient's arterial blood gas evaluation as things like the total CO2 level, base excess, and pH level all help determine the patient's status.

Indications: The arterial blood gas analysis and the bicarbonate level as part of this test is indicated for the evaluation of very sick patients who may have respiratory or metabolic disorders that have adversely affected the blood pH level and will cause disruption of the oxygenation and tissue metabolism unless the underlying cause of the disorder is identified and treated.

Normal Range: The normal arterial bicarbonate level is between 22 and 26 mmol/L.

Critical Range: There is no critical level for the arterial bicarbonate value.

Increased Value May Indicate: An elevated bicarbonate level associated with a high pH level in the arterial blood indicates metabolic alkalosis. Common causes of metabolic alkalosis include hypokalemia, chronic acid loss from vomiting, and an overdose of sodium bicarbonate.

Decreased Value May Indicate: A reduced bicarbonate level associated with a low pH in the arterial blood is indicative of metabolic acidosis.

The blood is too acidic for metabolic reasons, which can include shock, renal failure, and severe diabetic ketoacidosis.

Factors, Risks, or Other Information: An arterial blood gas measurement is technically difficult to obtain and is painful for the conscious patient. Complications can include a hematoma at the site of arterial blood retrieval if hemostasis isn't maintained for several minutes after taking the blood or if the patient has a bleeding disorder making it difficult to clot blood after an arterial puncture.

Acidity or Alkalinity of Blood

Abbreviation: pH

How Is It Measured: The blood pH is determined by doing an arterial blood gas assessment. Blood is taken from the radial or femoral artery into a heparinized syringe. All visible air bubbles are removed from the sample and the sample is placed on ice where it is kept until an urgent assessment of the arterial blood gas parameters can be obtained by a blood gas analyzer.

Description: The pH of the blood is the measurement of the balance between the acids and bases in the blood. It can be thrown off balance for metabolic or respiratory reasons. The body attempts to maintain a normal blood pH at all costs so, if the pH is abnormal, the typical mechanisms to restore a normal pH level in the arterial blood have been disrupted or haven't had time to take place.

Indications: The blood pH and the arterial blood gases are obtained in critically ill patients who have either respiratory dysfunction or metabolic dysfunction that have affected the amount of acids and bases in the bloodstream, throwing off the arterial blood pH. Normally, these are acute conditions as the body has mechanisms for restoring a normal pH balance over time, regardless of the cause.

Normal Range: The normal range for the arterial blood pH is 7.34 to 7.44.

Critical Range: A critically low arterial pH level is anything less than 7.22, while a critically high arterial pH level is anything higher than 7.59.

Increased Value May Indicate: An increased arterial blood pH level indicates either respiratory alkalosis or metabolic alkalosis. Causes of respiratory alkalosis include hyperventilation, certain lung diseases, or emotional distress. Causes of metabolic alkalosis include hypokalemia, sodium bicarbonate overdose, or losses of stomach acid from severe vomiting.

Decreased Value May Indicate: A decreased arterial blood pH level indicates either respiratory acidosis or metabolic acidosis. Causes of respiratory acidosis include underventilation and respiratory depression from sedation, pneumonia, and COPD. Causes of metabolic acidosis include diabetic ketoacidosis, renal failure, and shock.

Factors, Risks, or Other Information: Arterial blood gases are extremely painful to have done in the conscious patient and are technically difficult to obtain. The pH is just one aspect of the total picture, which can help identify an underlying cause for an acid-base abnormality, which can then be treated. The most common complication of an arterial gas measurement test is a hematoma at the site of the testing, which can be overcome by having strict hemostasis for several minutes after the test is taken. Patients with bleeding disorders are at a particularly high risk of having bleeding complications after an arterial blood gas measurement.

Oxygen Saturation

Abbreviation: O2 Sat

How Is It Measured: The oxygen saturation is a part of the arterial blood gas measurement. The patient has blood drawn from the radial or femoral artery under sterile technique. Arterial blood is drawn into a heparinized syringe and is placed on ice for urgent transfer to the laboratory for a blood gas analysis.

Description: The oxygen saturation level is included in the blood gas measurement. A rough approximation of the oxygen saturation can also be obtained in noninvasive ways by placing an O2 sat meter on the finger, ear lobes, or toes. This can read the oxygen saturation level in patients not requiring a full arterial blood gas measurement.

Indications: Patients will now routinely have a noninvasive O2 saturation level done using a finger probe when they are evaluated for any condition in the emergency department or in an outpatient clinic. The patient will have a full blood gas assessment of arterial blood if there is a question of low oxygen saturations from lung underventilation or underperfusion of the lungs or if there is evidence of an acid-base disorder.

Normal Range: The normal range for oxygen saturation is 95-100 percent saturation of arterial blood.

Critical Range: A critically low level of oxygen saturation is 90 percent or lower. There is no critically high oxygen saturation level.

Increased Value May Indicate: Patients with normal lung function can have oxygen saturation levels of 100 percent and this is completely normal. Ranges of 100 percent can also be seen in hyperventilation and in patients receiving oxygen therapy.

Decreased Value May Indicate: Decreased values can mean underperfusion of the lungs as can been seen in a pulmonary embolism. Low levels can be seen in underventilation states, which can be seen in a variety of lung diseases, including COPD, pneumonia, asthma, bronchitis, pneumothorax, and many other lung disorders.

Factors, Risks, or Other Information: The oxygen saturation level as gotten by finger probe carries no risk. If the oxygen saturation is gotten from an arterial blood gas measurement, the test can be technically difficult to do and is very painful. Complications include hematoma formation after the blood draw from a lack of adequate hemostasis for several minutes after retrieving the blood or from having a bleeding problem that interferes with the test.

Partial Pressure of Carbon Dioxide

Abbreviation: PaCO2

How Is It Measured: The partial pressure of carbon dioxide is a part of the arterial blood gas measurement. The patient has a sterile preparation of the skin over the brachial artery or femoral artery and blood is drawn from the artery into a heparinized syringe. The specimen is iced an urgently measured in a blood gas analyzer.

Description: The PaCO2 test is directly measured from the arterial blood gas measurement. It is an indicator of CO2 production by the body and the elimination of CO2 by the lungs. The PaCO2 is entirely determined by the lungs through ventilation.

Indications: Indications for the test include evaluation of very sick patients who may be underventilating or hyperventilating. Patients with suspected acid-base disorders have suspected PaO2 abnormalities that can be evaluated by checking the arterial blood gases and determining the partial pressure of carbon dioxide.

Normal Range: The normal range for PaCO2 is 35-45 mmHg

Critical Range: The critically low level for PaCO2 is anything less than 21 mmHg, while the upper critical value for PaCO2 is anything greater than 69 mmHg.

Increased Value May Indicate: Elevated PaCO2 levels can be seen in respiratory acidosis, which is generally caused by underventilation of the lungs, respiratory failure, and severe pulmonary diseases, such as COPD. This is also known as hypercapnia.

Decreased Value May Indicate: Low levels of PaCO2 can mean respiratory alkalosis. Patients who are hyperventilating acutely will have low PaCO2 levels because they are blowing of CO2. This disorder is also referred to as hypocapnia. Overventilation on mechanical ventilation can also mean a low partial pressure of carbon dioxide.

Factors, Risks, or Other Information: The main risk for obtaining the PaCO2 level is that it requires an arterial blood stick. Blood is taken from a heparinized syringe that has obtained arterial blood from a radial or femoral artery. The main complication of this is hematoma formation at the site of blood draw, which can be from a lack of adequate hemostasis after the procedure or from having a bleeding disorder that interferes with blood clotting.

Partial Pressure of Oxygen

Abbreviation: PaO2

How Is It Measured: The PaO2 is directly measured in an arterial blood gas sampling. Under sterile conditions, blood is obtained from the femoral or radial artery. Visible bubbled of air are removed and the specimen is placed on ice for an urgent measurement of the various blood gas components in a blood gas analyzer.

Description: The PaO2 is important in determining the PaO2 because it is a direct measure of how well the patient is oxygenating. It does not participate in acid-base measurements but can directly measure the patient's ability to oxygenate themselves with lung disease or acute lung problems.

Indications: If a patient has a low oxygen saturation on a finger probe, this may mean an underventilated or underperfused state that will need further evaluation with an arterial blood gas. Arterial blood gases can be done directly on critically ill patients to evaluate the status of their lungs.

Normal Range: The normal range for PaO2 is 80-100 mm Hg.

Critical Range: There is no critically high state for PaO2 levels; however, a critically low PaCO2 level is likely to be less than 51 mm Hg.

Increased Value May Indicate: Elevated levels of PaO2 can be seen in hyperventilation or in patients who are receiving supplemental oxygen or are on mechanical ventilation for various reasons.

Decreased Value May Indicate: Low PaO2 levels correlate with low oxygen saturation levels and represent underperfusion or underventilation of the lungs. This can be due to respiratory failure, pneumonia, COPD, tension pneumothorax, or sedation. A pulmonary embolism can also be a cause of low PaO2 levels.

Factors, Risks, or Other Information: This test is part of an arterial blood gas determinations, which can be a technically difficult test to perform. Major complications include hematoma formation at the site of the arterial puncture, which can be made worse if the patient has a bleeding disorder.

4.03 Complete Blood Count or CBC

This panel of lab values consists of:

- Basophils
- Eosinophils
- Monocytes
- Neutrophils
- Lymphocytes
- Reticulocytes
- Hematocrit
- Hemoglobin
- Red Blood Cell Count (RBC)
- Mean Corpuscular Hemoglobin
- Mean Corpuscular Hemoglobin Concentration
- Mean Corpuscular Volume
- White Blood Cell Count
- Platelet Count

Basophils

Abbreviation: Baso

How Is It Measured: The basophil count is one aspect of a complete blood cell count. It is done by obtaining venous blood through a lavender top tube, which contains EDTA to prevent blood clotting. The basophil count can be evaluated by means of a mechanical counter or from doing a peripheral smear and evaluation the number of basophils in the blood sample.

Description: Basophils are produced in the bone marrow and are the rarest type of white blood cell. The cell type is known as a granulocyte as there are granules in the cytoplasm of these cells. The main function of these types of cells is the release of substance from the granules that help kill foreign invaders.

Indications: There is no particular reason to order just a basophil level as it is part of a peripheral smear evaluation or an automated WBC count machine. If a patient has known basophilia from inflammation or cancer, this test can be used to follow it.

Normal Range: The normal range for the basophil count is 0.01-0.1 x 10^9 cells per liter or less than 2 percent.

Critical Range: The critical range for basophil count is anything greater than 2 percent in the peripheral smear evaluation.

Increased Value May Indicate: The most common reason for a high basophil count would be allergies. Rarer causes of a high basophil count include viral infections, Hodgkin lymphoma, CML, myelodysplastic syndrome, ulcerative colitis, Crohn's disease, low thyroid conditions, hemolytic anemia, parasitic infections chronic sinus infections, and surgical removal of the spleen.

Decreased Value May Indicate:

There is generally no problem with a low basophil count. Low counts can be seen in allergies that are extremely severe, pregnancy, corticosteroid use, or hyperthyroid states.

Factors, Risks, or Other Information: There is no risk in having the basophil count drawn. The test is interpreted as part of the various cells counted in a CBC. Because there are very few basophils, a count of 0 percent is not uncommon.

Eosinophils

Abbreviation: Eos

How Is It Measured: The eosinophil count is part of a manual or machine-generated count of the numbers of white blood cells in a sample of whole blood that is placed from a venipuncture into a lavender tube that contains EDTA. As the numbers of eosinophils are small, a peripheral smear is the best way to determine this value.

Description: The eosinophil count is counted by a peripheral smear and is check for when a patient is suspected of having allergies or inflammatory disorders. The test is usually done on a routine basis by an automated counter machine. If there is something abnormal in automated test, a peripheral smear can detect the level of eosinophils with greater accuracy. The eosinophil level is drawn when allergies, certain inflammatory disorders, drug reactions, parasitic infestations, and some cancers are suspected.

Indications: An automated eosinophil is determined as part of a routine CBC evaluation in a healthy individual. It can also be used to detect the presence of allergies, autoimmune disorders, inflammatory states, or in the evaluation and management of certain drug reactions, parasitic infections, and some cancers.

Normal Range: The normal range for the eosinophil count is 0.04 to 0.4 x 10^9 cells per liter or 0-6.0 percent.

Critical Range: As the eosinophil count is low, there is no critical lower limit for eosinophilia. The upper critical limit for the eosinophil count is anything greater than 6.0 percent.

Increased Value May Indicate: Eosinophilia may be seen with patients with allergic disorders. Skin diseases, medications, collagen-vascular diseases, malignancies or myeloproliferative diseases, parasitic infections, and bacterial infections. Any disease of the epithelial cells can result in eosinophilia.

Decreased Value May Indicate: As there are low numbers of eosinophils in the peripheral smear, a low level of eosinophils in the smear is usually a normal finding; however, persistently low levels can be seen myelofibrotic diseases of the bone marrow, which makes few or no white blood cells.

Factors, Risks, or Other Information: While eosinophilia is associated with allergies and certain infectious diseases (like parasitic disease), it can't be used to diagnose these disorders but is only a confirmatory finding.

Monocytes

Abbreviation: Mono

How Is It Measured: The monocyte level is part of a peripheral smear that is assessed by taking venous blood from a venipuncture, placing the blood in a lavender top tube. The monocyte can be counted with a cell counter or a peripheral smear can be obtained for a more accurate measurement of the monocyte count.

Description: The monocyte count is rarely checked alone but is part of a panel of white blood cells that are counted in a cell counter or in a peripheral smear count. The most accurate way of determining this level is the peripheral smear as the numbers of cells are low and the cell counter can be inaccurate.

Indications: The cell counter can check a monocyte count as part of a general health panel on healthy individuals. The test is not used to identify any particular disorder but can be a confirmatory test for parasitic infections, measles, or infectious mononucleosis.

Normal Range: The normal range for the monocyte count is 0.2 to 0.8 x 10^9 cells per liter or 4-10 percent of all WBCs.

Critical Range: The critical range for the upper limit of monocytes is called monocytosis and is any level greater than 15 percent.

Increased Value May Indicate: increased monocyte counts or monocytosis can be seen in infectious mononucleosis, leukemia, tuberculosis, measles, chronic inflammation, and mumps.

Decreased Value May Indicate: There are no diseases that are related to low monocyte counts. The absolute value of this white blood cell count is low already so lower levels than expected can be a normal variant. Rarely, a zero count of monocytes is related to bone marrow failure with low blood cell counts in all cell lines.

Factors, Risks, or Other Information: A monocyte count is not a diagnostic tool for any disease but is a confirmatory test that indicates the possible presence of any one of the causes of monocytosis. Further testing is necessary and will be more accurate in determining the exact cause of the monocytosis

Neutrophils

Abbreviation: Neut

How Is It Measured: The neutrophil count is part of a microscopic CBC evaluation. It is the most common type of leukocyte in peripheral blood so it is easy to count with a peripheral smear. The blood for evaluation comes from a venous blood draw and is placed into a lavender top tube. Whole blood can count the neutrophil level with a cell counter or manually, by obtaining a peripheral smear.

Description: Neutrophils represent the most common type of leukocyte. It is a good measurement for infectious diseases, particularly bacterial infections, as well as inflammation. A manual count with a peripheral smear is more accurate than a counted neutrophil count by a cell counter.

Indications: The neutrophil count can be part of a normal WBC count analysis in healthy individuals who can have the test done with a cell counter. A peripheral smear can be obtained to look for the absolute percentage of neutrophils and immature neutrophils, which are commonly seen in infectious disease, myeloproliferative diseases, and certain inflammatory diseases.

Normal Range: The normal range for the neutrophil count is 34-80 percent in healthy cells or 1.5 to 7.5K per microliter.

Critical Range: The critical range for the neutrophil count is any neutrophil percentage higher than 80 percent or greater than 7.9×10^9 cells per liter.

Increased Value May Indicate: increased neutrophil counts are also called neutrophilic leukocytosis or neutrophilia. The most common causes of neutrophilia include acute bacterial infections from any source or from a sterile inflammatory process, such as a crush injury, severe burns, or MI. Anytime active tissue repair is going on, the neutrophil count may be elevated. Chronic myelogenous leukemia can cause an absolute increase in neutrophils, which are primarily immature neutrophils being spilled out from the bone marrow.

Decreased Value May Indicate: Decreased white blood cells have several implications. Neutropenia, or a low white blood cell count, can mean a person is on chemotherapy, has HIV disease (although this usually affects the lymphocyte count), myelofibrosis or a leukemia involving another cell line, resulting in a decreased production of neutrophils in the bone marrow.

Factors, Risks, or Other Information: There are no particular risks for having this venipuncture test done. Unlike other white blood cell counts, the neutrophil count has several good applications for diagnostic purposes. An elevated white blood cell count can signify a bacterial infection, while a low white blood cell count can signify chemotherapy use, HIV disease, or myelofibrosis.

Lymphocytes

Abbreviation: Lymph

How Is It Measured: The lymphocyte count is measured electronically by a cell counter using a sample of venous blood that has been obtained in a venipuncture and from blood put into a lavender top tube with EDTA in it. If the count is abnormal or a more accurate level is necessary, the patient can have a peripheral smear done to manually measure the lymphocyte count.

Description: The lymphocyte count, obtained as above, has clinical implications in several diseases. It is usually best obtained by evaluating a peripheral smear in patient suspected of having a lymphocytic leukemia, a viral infection, HIV/AIDS disease,

Indications: A lymphocyte count can't diagnose a disease but can be seen anytime there is monocytosis in the blood. It is also elevated in various viral infections, such as cytomegalovirus, acute hepatitis, or any Epstein-Barr infection. In patients with a severe cough, a lymphocyte can be evaluated to see if the patient has Bordetella pertussis.

Normal Range: The normal range for the lymphocyte count is 1.0-3.0 x 10^9 cells per liter or 20-40 percent of all leukocytes.

Critical Range: The critical low level of the lymphocyte count is 1.0 x 10^9 cells per liter, while the critical level for a high level of lymphocytes or lymphocytosis is anything above 3.5 x 10^9 cells per liter.

Increased Value May Indicate: Increased levels of lymphocytes are commonly seen in a variety of viral diseases, such as cytomegalovirus, Epstein-Barr virus, influenza, and hepatitis. It can also be seen in Bordetella pertussis infections (whooping cough) and in myeloproliferative disorders and cancers, such as acute lymphocytic leukemia or chronic lymphocytic leukemia. Smoking can increase the lymphocyte level.

Decreased Value May Indicate: The T lymphocyte count is particularly low in HIV/AIDS, where the T helper cell level or CD4 cell level can be critically low. The cell count can be also low in bone marrow disorders that aren't making any cell lines or that are making some cell lines in excess, with low levels of lymphocytes made. Humoral immune deficiency can result in a decrease in B lymphocytes. The most common cause of lymphopenia is the common cold and other infections that temporarily suppress the lymphocyte count.

Factors, Risks, or Other Information: There are no risks to having a lymphocyte count drawn. The test is a suggestive test, meaning that it can suggest the presence of disease but can't diagnose a disease unless further testing is performed.

Reticulocytes

Abbreviation: Retic count

How Is It Measured: The reticulocyte count is measured by doing a venipuncture and placing whole blood in a lavender (EDTA) tube, which is then placed into a cell counter. The reticulocyte count is measured in the counter.

Description: The reticulocyte count is a direct measure of erythropoiesis. When more red blood cells, in particular, immature red blood cells called reticulocytes, are released from the bone marrow, more of these cells can be seen in the peripheral circulation, indicating that red blood cells are being made.

Indications: The main reason for doing a reticulocyte count is to measure the number of red blood cells being put out by the bone marrow. In certain types of anemia, such as iron deficiency anemia, the reticulocyte count will be elevated, distinguishing it from other types of microcytic anemia.

Normal Range: The normal range for the reticulocyte count is 0.5 to 1.5 percent.

Critical Range: There are no critical values for high or low reticulocyte counts. Elevated counts just mean increased erythropoiesis, which isn't a clinical problem but a sign of another disease.

Increased Value May Indicate: Increased reticulocyte counts basically mean enhanced erythropoiesis from various anemic states, such as blood loss anemia, hemolytic anemia, thalassemia, sideroblastic anemia, bone transplant patients, and patients begin treated for iron deficiency anemia.

Decreased Value May Indicate: Low lab values of the reticulocyte count mean that the bone marrow isn't putting out a lot of immature red blood cells as can be seen in aplastic anemia or in an aplastic crisis in patients with hemolytic anemia.

Factors, Risks, or Other Information: The reticulocyte count is not a risky test to do. It can be detected in an automatic cell counter but is a much more accurate test when evaluated manually with a peripheral smear because these represent nucleated red blood cells that can accidentally be labeled as a leukocyte on the cell analyzer.

Hematocrit

Abbreviation: HCT or Hct or Crit

How Is It Measured: The hematocrit is part of a whole blood profile that includes a hemoglobin, hematocrit, RBC level, WBCs, and indices. It is collected by means of a venipuncture in a lavender top tube; whole blood is electronically evaluated with the hematocrit being electronically calculated.

Description: The hematocrit test is one of a couple of tests for anemia and usually trends along with the hemoglobin level, both of which are a part of a CBC evaluation. The test can screen for anemia, diagnose blood disorders, and can monitor the results of treatment for an elevated hematocrit or a low hematocrit.

Indications: The major indications for a hematocrit include evaluating the severity of anemia or high hematocrit states, such as polycythemia. The response to therapy can be evaluated with this test. This test can identify patients who need blood transfusions or patients who might have high hematocrit levels from being dehydrated. Bone marrow diseases that result in a reduction in the number of RBCs being released into the bloodstream will reveal themselves initially as a low hematocrit. While it is a good screening test for red blood cell diseases, it cannot diagnose the cause of the problem and further testing is usually required to actually diagnose the problem.

Normal Range: The normal hematocrit level in adult males is 41.5 percent to 50.4 percent, while the normal hematocrit for adult females is 36.9 percent to 44.6 percent.

Critical Range: A critical range for hematocrit is less than 21 percent or greater than 55 percent.

Increased Value May Indicate: Increased hematocrit levels are usually associated with polycythemia or too many red blood cells. Common causes are dehydration, certain lung diseases with hypoxemia, birth defects of the heart with hypoxemia, smoking history, living in a high altitude, or having polycythemia vera.

Decreased Value May Indicate: Low hematocrit levels usually mean low red blood cell counts with anemia. Common causes of anemia include chronic blood loss, iron deficiency, deficiencies in the absorption of vitamin B12 or folate, damage to bone marrow from chemotherapy or radiation, kidney failure with decreased erythropoietin levels, hemoglobinopathies, and hemolytic anemia.

Factors, Risks, or Other Information: The hematocrit level will not reflect an accurate measure of the patient's blood status if they recently had a blood transfusion. Due to extra fluid volume expansion, the hematocrit in pregnancy is low. There are no risks to having a hematocrit level evaluated.

Hemoglobin

Abbreviation: HGB or Hgb or H

How Is It Measured: The hemoglobin measurement is obtained by doing a venipuncture and placing the blood in a lavender top tube that contains EDTA. The blood is placed in a cell counter and a hemoglobin level is calculated from this testing.

Description: Hemoglobin is often tested if there is clinical suspicion of anemia. It can be tested alone but can be tested as part of a complete blood count, which includes the hematocrit. It can screen for various diseases that affect the red blood cell count and hemoglobin level. Hemoglobin is a protein that carries iron and oxygen in red blood cells and is best interpreted along with red blood cell indices and the hematocrit.

Indications: The hemoglobin test can be done on normal individuals as part of normal screening. It can diagnose and interpret the severity of various anemias as well as polycythemia (which is an elevation of hemoglobin and RBCs in the blood). Treatment response to these diseases can be done by reevaluating the hemoglobin. Patients needing a transfusion can be identified by checking a hemoglobin. Clinical signs that might indicate a need for a hemoglobin include fatigue, low energy levels, shortness of breath, pale skin, and syncope. Clinical signs of polycythemia include headache, poor vision, dizziness, enlargement of the spleen, and facial flushing.

Normal Range: The normal hemoglobin range in adult men is 14-17.5 g/dL, while the normal hemoglobin range for females is 12.3 to 15.3 g/dL.

Critical Range: The low critical value for hemoglobin is less than 7 g/dL, while the upper critical level for hemoglobin is greater than 18 g/dL.

Increased Value May Indicate: High levels of hemoglobin associated with a high RBC count and a high hematocrit is usually secondary to polycythemia. Some causes of this include birth defects of the heart, lung disease, benign kidney adenomas, smoking, dehydration, high altitudes, and a rare disease called polycythemia vera.

Decreased Value May Indicate: Low levels of hemoglobin associated with a low RBC count and a low hematocrit are due to anemia of many causes. Some include chronic bleeding, iron deficiency anemia, B12 or folate anemia, bone marrow dysfunction, severe kidney failure, abnormal hemoglobinopathies, and chronic inflammation.

Factors, Risks, or Other Information: Patients with a recent transfusion of blood will have an improvement in their hemoglobin level. A normal hemoglobin in pregnancy is lower that the hemoglobin outside of pregnancy.

Red Blood Cell Count

Abbreviation: RBC

How Is It Measured: A red blood cell count is a measure of the concentration of red blood cells in whole blood. Blood is collected by means of a venipuncture and placed in a lavender top tube. The blood is evaluated as whole blood by a red blood cell counter, which also evaluates the white blood cell count, hematocrit, and hemoglobin levels. RBC indices are also measured in this test.

Description: A red blood cell count or RBC count is part of a total CBC test. It can be used as a screening test to evaluate the patient for several different medical conditions. It detects problems with either the production of red blood cells or the lifespan of the red blood cells. Normal RBCs have a 120-day lifespan but if this is shortened for any reason, the RBC will be less. There are also diseases affecting the number of RBCs made by the bone marrow and this can affect the RBC count. Sometimes, RBCs can be deformed and can have a shorter lifespan, which can affect the total count.

Indications: The RBC count is ordered not as a separate test but is done as part of the CBC evaluation. It is indicated for evidence of anemia, such as tiredness, poor energy, or pale skin. Signs of elevated RBC levels include visual disturbances, facial flushing, splenic enlargement, dizziness, and headache. Other indications of checking the RBC level is to monitor the treatment given for high RBC states or low RBC states.

Normal Range: The normal range for an RBC count is 4.5 to 5.9×10^6 cells per microliter in adult males, while the normal range for an RBC count is $4.5-5.1 \times 10^6$ cells per microliter in adult females.

Critical Range: A critically low red blood cell count is less than 3.0×10^6 cells per microliter, while a critically high red blood cell count is greater than 6.0×10^6 cells per microliter.

Increased Value May Indicate: Causes of high RBC levels or polycythemia include dehydration (with plasma loss compared to blood counts), lung diseases with hypoxia, congenital heart diseases with hypoxia, kidney tumors that make erythropoietin, polycythemia vera, or genetic diseases.

Decreased Value May Indicate: Red blood cell loss from hemorrhage or bone marrow failure will decrease the RBC count. Things that might come into play include traumatic injury, hemolytic anemia, hemoglobinopathies, chronic bleeding nutritional deficiencies, or bone marrow failure. Sometimes the bone marrow can be involved in making too many other cell lines, causing a deficiency in making the RBC cell line. Kidney failure with reduced erythropoietin levels will result in low RBC levels.

Factors, Risks, or Other Information: The treatment for a low RBC count is a blood transfusion if the RBC count reaches critically low values. When the RBC count is found to be abnormal, this does not diagnose disease but will lead the healthcare professional to further evaluate the patient. The reason why RBC levels are higher at high altitudes is that there is an excess need for oxygen at elevated altitudes.

Mean Corpuscular Hemoglobin

Abbreviation: MCH

How Is It Measured: The MCH level is simply an attribute of the red blood cell so it is determined as part of a red blood cell determination. Blood Is taken from a venipuncture and placed in a lavender top tube. Whole blood is measured, including the hemoglobin, hematocrit, RBC level, and indices, of which the MCH is one of them.

Description: The MCH test is measured mechanically and is a measurement of the mean corpuscular hemoglobin level in each red blood cell. Some cells have a lot of hemoglobin in them, while other red blood cells are either smaller or paler, having a low mean corpuscular hemoglobin level.

Indications: The only real indication for the mean corpuscular hemoglobin level is as part of an assessment of the characteristics of the RBC. The MCH, MCHC, and MCV are used together to identify the size of the red blood cells in the individual's blood stream and the amount of hemoglobin found each cell. It is done to identify the type of anemia or red blood cell abnormality the patient has.

Normal Range: The normal MCH level is 27.5-33.2 pg in both men and women.

Critical Range: There is no critical level of MCH that needs clinical attention.

Increased Value May Indicate: An elevated MCH level may mean that the RBCs are large and therefore contain a great deal of hemoglobin. Small or normal cells may have a high concentration of hemoglobin so the MCH must be evaluated along with the MCV and the MCHC level to make a determination of the characteristics of the cells.

Decreased Value May Indicate: Decreased MCH levels may mean that the patient has very small cells that don't contain a great deal of hemoglobin in them. It also may mean that the patient has normal-sized

RBCs or large RBCs that are pale in appearance because they have low concentrations of hemoglobin and low total MCH levels.

Factors, Risks, or Other Information: The MCH test alone says very little about the individual's red blood cells until the test is compared along with and MCHC test and an MCV test, which can help identify the type of red blood cell abnormality a patient has.

Mean Corpuscular Hemoglobin Concentration

Abbreviation: MCHC

How Is It Measured: The mean corpuscular hemoglobin concentration or MCHC is measured by testing whole blood obtained from a venipuncture. The whole blood is temporarily stored in a lavender top tube and then is run through a whole blood analyzer, which detects the RBCs, WBCs, and platelets, along with the various characteristics of these types of cells.

Description: The mean corpuscular hemoglobin concentration is the concentration of hemoglobin in the cells irrespective of the size of the cells. In a very real sense, it is a measurement of how pale or how red the blood cells look as cells with a greater concentration of hemoglobin in them will have a higher MCHC.

Indications: The main indications for doing an MCHC on an RBC evaluation is to determine the characteristics of the red blood cells. The mean corpuscular hemoglobin concentration says a lot about how much hemoglobin is packed in each cell. Situations where large oxygen transfers are necessary will have a larger concentration of hemoglobin in each cell. The MCHC, however, says nothing about the size of the cell and is therefore only a part of the evaluation of the probable cause of anemia the patient has.

Normal Range: The normal range for the MCHC is 33.4-35.5 g/dL in both males and females.

Critical Range: There are no critical values for the MCHC that are clinically important or designated.

Increased Value May Indicate: Increased MCHC concentrations are extremely rare but can be seen in autoimmune hemolytic anemia patients, patients with severe burns, and patients with hereditary spherocytosis.

Decreased Value May Indicate: Decreased MCHC concentrations usually mean the cells are pale and there is a lack of substrate to make hemoglobin for the cells. Low MCHC concentrations are seen in iron deficiency anemia and thalassemia.

Factors, Risks, or Other Information: The mean corpuscular hemoglobin concentration is not capable of diagnosing the type of anemia or polycythemia the patient has as it needs to be compared directly with the MCV and the MCH to better understand the size and other characteristics of the cell.

Mean Corpuscular Volume

Abbreviation: MCV

How Is It Measured: The mean corpuscular volume is one of three RBC indices that are determined at the time of an RBC evaluation. It is measured from whole blood obtained from a venipuncture and is stored in a lavender top tube until it is evaluated in a whole blood analyzer, which measures the RBCs, platelets, and WBCs, as well as the characteristics of the RBCs, of which the MCV is one of them.

Description: The mean corpuscular volume is a direct measurement of the size of red blood cells in a whole blood sample. Cells that are large, such as is seen in macrocytic anemia, will have a large MCV, while cells that are small, such as is seen in iron deficiency anemia, will have a low MCV.

Indications: Red blood cell indices, such as the MCV, are ordered as part of the CBC evaluation and are used to attempt to measure the hemoglobin in the cells as it relates to the size of the cells. The MCV, MCHC, and MCH together are used to evaluate the qualities of the red blood cell as they are important in identifying the type of RBC disorder the patient has.

Normal Range: The normal range for the MCV is 80-96 micrometer^3 for both adult males and adult females.

Critical Range: There is no critical range for the MCV that is important for clinical purposes.

Increased Value May Indicate: An elevated mean corpuscular volume means that the RBCs are larger than normal and are considered macrocytic cells. This can be seen in a variety of blood and non-blood-related diseases, such as B12 deficiency, folate deficiency, liver disease, low thyroid conditions, and myelodysplasia.

Decreased Value May Indicate: Decreased MCV levels mean that the red blood cells are smaller than normal and are considered microcytic.

Common microcytic blood diseases are thalassemia and iron deficiency anemia.

Factors, Risks, or Other Information: The mean cell volume or MCV alone is not sufficient to make an adequate determination of the type of blood disorder the patient has. It needs to be compared with the MCH and the MCHC in order to attempt to understand the total characteristics of the RBC.

White Blood Cell Count

Abbreviation: WBC

How Is It Measured: The white blood cell count is a part of a CBC evaluation and is taken from whole blood. The blood is obtained by a venipuncture and is stored in and EDTA-containing lavender top tube, where it is then run in a whole blood cell counter that measures the WBC level, the platelet level, and the RBC level. A breakdown of the types of WBCs in the specimen can also be made with an automatic counter.

Description: The WBCs are the immune cells of the body and these are measured as part of the CBC evaluation. The WBC count is an important aspect of this evaluation as it can determine if the patient has an infection, inflammation in the body, or an abnormal state of having too little WBCs in the body.

Indications: The WBC count is measured to see if there is infection, leukemia, lymphomas, or inflammation in the body. The total WBC count isn't as important as the breakdown of WBCs as different disorders will have different levels of lymphocytes, monocytes, neutrophils, eosinophils, and basophils in the blood.

Normal Range: The normal range for the WBC count is 4,500-11,000 white blood cells per microliter (mcL) for both adult men and adult women.

Critical Range: The critical range for the upper and lower WBC limit for both adult men and adult women is less than 1,500 cells per microliter or more than 30,000 cells per microliter.

Increased Value May Indicate: Elevated levels of the white blood cell count is known as leukocytosis. The most common reason for this is a viral or bacterial infection. Inflammation in the body can raise the WBC level and patients with myeloproliferative disorders or leukemia will have elevated WBC levels. Allergies and asthma can raise WBC levels. High WBC levels can be seen in extreme stress, intense exercise, severe burns, a heart attack, or major trauma situations with tissue death.

Decreased Value May Indicate: A low WBC level is known as leukopenia. Bone marrow disorders or damage to the bone marrow can result in a lack of WBC production and leukopenia. Severe infections, such as sepsis, will actually decrease the WBC level. Patients with cancers to bone, such as lymphomas, will make certain blood cell lines but will not make other cell lines, resulting in leukopenia. Patients with HIV/AIDS have disordered immune systems and will not make helper T cells, resulting in an overall low WBC value.

Factors, Risks, or Other Information: Low WBC values or high WBC values will not be sufficient on their own to determine the cause of the person's problem. The type of WBC is just as important as the total number of WBCs so the differential done electronically or manually will help define the type of problem the patient is having.

Platelet Count

Abbreviation: Plat

How Is It Measured: The platelet count is part of the CBC evaluation, which is taken from whole blood can be determined by taking a venous sample that is stored in a lavender top tube containing EDTA and that is placed as whole blood into a whole blood cell counter, which can measure the WBC count, platelet count, and RBC count at once. The platelets are the smallest cellular components and the only thing measured as part of the evaluation of these cells is the total number.

Description: Platelets are important to the coagulation process, which is actually a complex process involving platelets and proteins that allow platelets to aggregate. The platelet count is measured as part of the CBC and is helpful but not necessarily diagnostic in determining if a patient has a problem with clotting.

Indications: The platelet count is sometimes evaluated before surgery to make sure that the patient has adequate platelets to clot blood before surgery. It is also done when a patient is suspected of having a bleeding disorder or if they seem to have an abnormally high propensity for clotting, even though the platelet count is just one measurement of many that go into the evaluation of an individual's clotting ability.

Normal Range: The normal range for the platelet count in adult males and females is 150,000 to 450,000 cells per microliter.

Critical Range: The critical range for the platelet count is less than 20,000 cells per microliter or greater than 1,000,000 cells per microliter.

Increased Value May Indicate: An elevated platelet count is known as thrombocytosis. There are many reasons for thrombocytosis including certain cancers, such as lymphomas, ovarian cancer, breast cancer, GI cancers, and lung cancer, which produce substances that promote platelet production. Platelets are also found to be elevated in SLE, inflammatory bowel disease, and rheumatoid arthritis. Iron deficiency anemia and hemolytic anemia will trigger an elevated platelet count. Patients with essential thrombocytopenia have a myeloproliferative disorder that results in a high bone marrow production of thrombocytes.

Decreased Value May Indicate: Low levels of platelets are also referred to as having thrombocytopenia. A low platelet count can be seen in certain infections, such as hepatitis, measles, and infectious mononucleosis. Rocky mountain spotted fever is another infectious disease associated with thrombocytopenia. Patients with autoantibodies to platelets will have a low platelet count and patients with any type of autoimmune disorder will exhibit thrombocytopenia. Sepsis, acetaminophen use, quinidine use, and the use of sulfa drugs may precipitate a low platelet count. Patients with cirrhosis can also have a low platelet count. Cancer patients on chemotherapy will not make very many platelets and will have a low platelet count.

Factors, Risks, or Other Information: There is no risk to having a platelet count drawn. It is important to remember that the platelet count is just one factor in the determination of a person's clotting ability. There are clotting factors and other proteins that contribute to the clotting process so a full determination of a person's ability to clot blood will require more than just the platelet determination.

4.04 Coagulation Profile Testing

The panel of lab values consists of:

- Prothrombin Time

- Partial Thromboplastin Time (PTT)

- International Normalized Ratio (INR)

Prothrombin Time

Abbreviation: PT or Protime

How Is It Measured: The protime is measured on venous blood as part of a panel of coagulation studies that can help evaluate an individual's ability to clot blood. Blood is taken from a peripheral vein and is placed in a light blue top tube containing sodium citrate to prevent clotting. The protime is measured along with other coagulation profile studies to fully evaluate a patient's clotting ability.

Description: The prothrombin time or PT is often checked along with the partial thromboplastin time or PTT in the evaluation of possible bleeding disorders. As the PT can vary according to the laboratory doing the testing, this value has been converted to the INR or international normalized ratio, which is a better assessment of bleeding that can be compared from laboratory to laboratory and is used to determine the effectiveness of warfarin in thinning the blood. The protime is actually a determination of the function of several coagulation factors involved in the coagulation process.

Indications: The prothrombin time and the INR are together used to determine how effective the anticoagulant, warfarin, is working to slow the clotting process. Warfarin does not act on the platelets but instead acts on several of the coagulation proteins that help platelets form thrombi. Patients on warfarin must ride a fine balance between clotting too much and bleeding too much so the protime and INR are calculated to make sure this balance is maintained.

Patients take warfarin for a variety of reasons, including atrial fibrillation or other cardiac arrhythmia, having an artificial heart valve, having a deep vein thrombosis or pulmonary embolism, having antiphospholipid syndrome, or recovering from a myocardial infarction or stroke.

In some cases, the prothrombin time can be evaluated along with the partial thromboplastin time to investigate excessive bleeding or excessive clotting disorders. The prothrombin time is a direct measurement of the function of the coagulation factors VII, X, VI, II, and I. The platelet count, the PT and the PTT are necessary evaluations to see what a person's clotting features are and the evaluation of the protime alone is insufficient to make a satisfactory diagnosis.

Normal Range: The normal range for a prothrombin time is 10.0-13.0 seconds.

Critical Range: There is actually no critical range for the prothrombin time. Instead, the prothrombin time is reinterpreted as the INR or international normalized ratio that will be discussed later. This value, the INR, does have a critical range that is indirectly related to the prothrombin time.

Increased Value May Indicate: For individuals who take warfarin, the protime is not reported but the INR Is instead the value reported. An INR of between 2.0 and 3.0 is considered optimal for patients taking this drug. The protime is measured in seconds and varies from laboratory to laboratory so the INR is what is reported. The protime can also be elevated in patients having certain clotting factor deficiencies, many of which are congenital deficiencies.

Decreased Value May Indicate: There really is no clinical disorder related to having a low prothrombin time. The prothrombin time is either normal or prolonged, with a prolonged prothrombin time having clinical significance. A low prothrombin time has no clinical significance.

Factors, Risks, or Other Information: The absolute value of the prothrombin time is less important than the international normalized ration or INR, which is calculated from the prothrombin time. Most laboratories report the INR when assessing the effectiveness of warfarin or when discussing the risk of abnormal bleeding in a patient with a bleeding disorder.

Partial Thromboplastin Time or Activated Partial Thromboplastin Time

Abbreviation: PTT or aPTT

How Is It Measured: The partial thromboplastin time or PTT and the activated partial thromboplastin time or aPTT are just a part of coagulation studies that are often done together to evaluate patients with clotting problems or, in the case of the PTT and aPTT, to evaluate patients on heparin. Whole venous blood is drawn from a peripheral vein and is placed in a light blue top tube containing sodium citrate. The PTT and aPTT are determined by the laboratory and is reported in seconds.

Description: The partial thromboplastin time is used to investigate cases where an individual has an unknown clotting disorder. In such cases, a prothrombin time is drawn, as well as a platelet count. The partial thromboplastin time does not evaluate the platelets but instead evaluates the function of the coagulation factors XI, XII, IX, VIII, X, II, I, and V. Because it does not evaluate all of the coagulation factors, the prothrombin time must be assessed along with this test. The PTT and the activated PTT or aPTT are basically the same test, except that the aPTT test has an activator added to the blood to speed up the clotting process so it has a narrower reference range.

Indications: There are several reasons why an individual might have a PTT drawn. They may be suspected of having a coagulation factor deficiency or dysfunction of a coagulation factor. Antibodies to coagulation factors can adversely affect the PTT. Nonspecific autoantibodies, such as those seen in patients with lupus, will have clotting excesses and recurrent miscarriages associated with abnormalities of their PTT. The PTT is also used to evaluate patients taking heparin intravenously to see if the heparin dose is adequate to prevent clotting. Patients will have both the prothrombin time and the partial thromboplastin time drawn if they have unexplained clotting or bleeding, disseminated intravascular coagulation, or chronic liver disease, in which the liver does not make enough clotting factors. Women who have lupus anticoagulant, antiphospholipid syndrome, or anticardiolipin antibodies will have recurrent miscarriages and need a prothrombin time and partial thromboplastin time evaluated. Patients having surgery will have a PTT evaluated to make sure their blood will clot during surgery.

Normal Range: The normal range for the aPTT is 28.5-37.5 seconds.

Critical Range: The critical range for the aPTT is any value greater than 150 seconds.

Increased Value May Indicate: A prolonged PTT can be seen in patients with inherited factor deficiencies, such as von Willebrand disease, which is the most commonly inherited clotting factor deficiency. Hemophilia A patients and hemophilia B patients will have abnormally high partial thromboplastin times. Acquired coagulation factor deficiencies, such as is seen with patients who have vitamin K deficiency will have both a prolonged PT and a prolonged PTT. Patients with lupus anticoagulant will have a long PTT and patients on intravenous heparin will have a prolonged PTT. Warfarin will prolong the PTT but this level is not used to monitor the drug's effectiveness. There are other, more rare anticoagulants, such as rivaroxaban, that will prolong the PTT. Patients with leukemia will have longer partial thromboplastin times.

Decreased Value May Indicate: It is possible to have a PTT that is too short; however, this is less common. It can be seen in disseminated intravascular coagulation, particularly in the early stages. Patients with severe colon, pancreatic, or ovarian cancers will have a shorter PTT. Patients with acute trauma or acute tissue inflammation will have a low PTT. After the acute phase has resolved, the PTT will normalize.

Factors, Risks, or Other Information: There are no risks in have the PTT or aPTT drawn, although patients with bleeding disorders may need to have prolonged pressure placed on the venipuncture site in order to make sure there is no excessive bleeding after having the test drawn. There are several reasons why a PTT might be artificially prolonged. Patients who have elevated hematocrit levels will have a prolonged PTT as will patients who have intravenous lines that have been contaminated with heparin. Patients taking vitamin C, chlorpromazine, aspirin, and antihistamines might have an artificially elevated PTT.

International Normalized Ratio

Abbreviation: INR

How Is It Measured: The international normalized ratio or INR is actually a calculated value based on the prothrombin time. The prothrombin time or PT is evaluated as part of a coagulation profile that includes the taking of venous blood through a peripheral vein and placing the blood in a light blue top tube with sodium citrate in it. The blood is measured as to its ability to clot over time and the INR is calculated so that the PT can be better correlated between laboratories and over a prolonged period of time.

Description: The INR is a completely calculated number that has no units. It accounts for differences in reagents and differences in the prothrombin times found in different populations of people. It is a better way of comparing the effects of warfarin on patients with clotting disorders.

Indications: The INR is almost exclusively measured in patients who have their prothrombin time assessed while they are on warfarin. Rather than trying to compare the PT between two different laboratories or over a long period of time, the INR was invented to makes sure the comparisons between blood draws of the individual's clotting ability can be assessed without having to account for variations between reagents and laboratories.

Normal Range: The normal range for the INR is 0.9-1.1. There are no units associated with the INR. Patients on warfarin are tried to maintain an INR of between 1.5 and 2.0.

Critical Range: The critical range for the INR is greater than 5.0.

Increased Value May Indicate: An increased value of INR means that the individual is on too high a dose of warfarin and needs a dosage adjustment. As long as the INR is not in the critical range, this can be accomplished by withholding the warfarin for a few days, reassessing the INR and starting the drug at a lower dose with more careful monitoring.

Decreased Value May Indicate: There is no such thing as a decreased INR. The normal range of about 1.0 is about as low as an INR can get with no clinical significance associated with having an INR much less than this.

Factors, Risks, or Other Information: There is no risk to having the INR evaluated as it is a calculated test. It has vastly improved the way warfarin patients are managed between laboratories and over time so that the drug can effectively be kept within the acceptable range as long as the patient is taking the drug.

4.05 Cholesterol Panel or Lipid Profile
The panel of lab values consists of:

- Total Cholesterol
- Low Density Lipoprotein
- High Density Lipoprotein
- Triglycerides

Total Cholesterol

Abbreviation: TChol

How Is It Measured: The total cholesterol is done as part of a lipid profile. It is done on serum separated from the blood components in a red top, red/gold top, or gold top tube after being drawn from a peripheral vein. A chemical analyzer evaluates the total cholesterol. The test is ideally done fasting as eating can artificially raise this blood level.

Description: The total cholesterol can be drawn as a single test or as part of a lipid profile that is ordinarily done to predict a person's chances of developing cardiovascular disease. Patients found to be at risk will often take medications to lower their risk by lowering their total and LDL cholesterol levels. High total cholesterol levels are associated with an increased risk of heart disease, cerebrovascular disease, and peripheral vascular disease so routine testing of normal adults is recommended. The results of the total cholesterol are compared to the results of other lipid studies to completely evaluate the patient's risk and to treat them accordingly.

Indications: Cholesterol testing is recommended as a screening tool for all adults, regardless of their clinical risk for heart disease, and for selected children and teens at a high risk for heart disease. The test should be done approximately every 4-6 years during a routine physical examination. Patients with major risk factors, such as tobacco use, obesity, poor dietary habits, sedentary lifestyle, diabetes, hypertension, positive family history of heart disease, or advanced age, should be tested more often.

Normal Range: A normal range for an adult having a total cholesterol reading on a fasting basis is less than 200 mg/dL.

Critical Range: Rather than having critical ranges for total cholesterol, patients are stratified according to their risk for heart disease. Patients who have total cholesterol levels of less than 200 mg/dL are considered to have a normal risk for heart disease. Patients with a total cholesterol of between 240 and 280 mg/dL have a high risk for heart disease, while patients with a total cholesterol of greater than 280 mg/dL have a very high risk for heart disease.

Increased Value May Indicate: As mentioned above, the total cholesterol level is stratified according to risk factor. A desirable total cholesterol is below 200 mg/dL. A borderline high cholesterol of between 200 and 239 mg/dL have a moderately high risk for heart disease. Patients with a total cholesterol of 240 to 279 mg/dL have a high risk for heart disease, while patients with a total cholesterol level of greater than 250 mg/dL are at a very high risk for heart disease.

Decreased Value May Indicate: There really aren't any clinical disorders associated with a low cholesterol. Some people who are extremely malnourished or very thin will have a reduced total cholesterol level. Patients with cancer will have low cholesterol levels but there isn't any evidence that this is harmful to the patient.

Factors, Risks, or Other Information: The total cholesterol level shouldn't be measured when a person is acutely ill as this can temporarily lower their total cholesterol. People under stress, who've had trauma, or who've had a heart attack are poor candidates to have a total cholesterol drawn as it will not accurately reflect their cholesterol level when they are well. In the same way, cholesterol levels are particularly high in pregnancy and don't reflect an added risk for heart disease. Patients who take vitamin D, epinephrine, oral contraceptives, or anabolic steroids may have elevated total cholesterol levels.

Low Density Lipoprotein

Abbreviation: LDL or LDL-c

How Is It Measured: The low-density lipoprotein test is part of the lipid profile drawn on fasting patients from a sampling of venous blood. The blood is stored in a red top, red/gold top, or gold top tube and is centrifuged until the serum is separated from the blood components. The serum is then electronically tested for the LDL-cholesterol level.

Description: The test for LDL-cholesterol is just one part of the lipid profile used to predict a person's overall risk of developing cardiovascular disease and to decide which patients will require lipid-lowering therapy to reduce their heart disease risk. LDL-C is not a directly measured laboratory value but is calculated from some of the other components of the lipid profile. For this reason, it is rarely ordered as a single test. High triglyceride levels can render the LDL-C test inaccurate. If this is the case, there is a directly measured LDL-C test available. LDL-cholesterol represents the single highest determinant of cardiovascular risk and is what people consider the "bad" cholesterol level. It is considered bad because it results in the deposition of cholesterol deposits on the inner lining of the major arteries.

Indications: The LDL-C level is done as part of a routine health examination in patients without risk factors for heart disease every 4-6 years. It should be done more frequently in patients who have cardiovascular risk factors, such as tobacco abuse, obesity, poor dietary habits, a sedentary lifestyle, hypertension, a positive family history of heart disease, older age, preexisting heart disease, or diabetes. The LDL-cholesterol level is ordered when a person is on a lipid-lowering medication along with dietary and exercise measures to make sure the medications are effective. It should be done 4-12 weeks after starting treatment and every 3-12 months after that.

Normal Range: The most desirable range for LDL-cholesterol is less than 100 mg/dL.

Critical Range: There is no critical range for LDL-cholesterol but instead patients are stratified according to their risk factors for heart disease. LDL-C levels between 130 and 159 mg/dL are considered borderline high; LDL-C levels between 160 and 189 mg/dL are considered high risk; and LDL-C levels above 190 mg/d: are considered very high risk.

Increased Value May Indicate: Among healthy individuals with no evidence of heart disease, the decision to treat the cholesterol levels alone must be weighed against the other risk factors the patient has for heart disease. Patients believed to have a 7.5 percent or higher risk for cardiovascular disease should be placed on statin drug therapy. A target reduction in the percentage of LDL-C from the baseline is considered a better approach than trying to reach an absolute value. Besides statin drugs, patients are encouraged to make lifestyle changes to attempt to reduce their LDL-C as much as possible.

Decreased Value May Indicate: Low LDL-cholesterol levels are unassociated with clinical problems and are not of a concern. It can be seen in patients with a genetic lipoprotein deficiency, in cirrhosis, in inflammatory conditions, in infections, and in individuals with hyperthyroidism.

Factors, Risks, or Other Information: The LDL-cholesterol level shouldn't be measured when a person is acutely ill as this can temporarily lower their LDL-cholesterol. People under stress, who've had trauma, or who've had a heart attack are poor candidates to have an LDL-cholesterol drawn as it will not accurately reflect their cholesterol level when they are well. In the same way, LDL-cholesterol levels are particularly high in pregnancy and don't reflect an added risk for heart disease. LDL-testing should wait until after the pregnancy has passed for at least six weeks.

High Density Lipoprotein

Abbreviation: HDL or HDL-C

How Is It Measured: The high-density lipoprotein test is part of the lipid profile drawn on fasting patients from a sampling of venous blood. The blood is stored in a red top, red/gold top, or gold top tube and is centrifuged until the serum is separated from the blood components. The serum is then electronically tested for the HDL-cholesterol level.

Description: The HDL-cholesterol test is generally not ordered alone but is done as part of a lipid profile in an attempt to screen healthy patients for an increased risk of heart disease based on abnormal lipid studies. The HDL-cholesterol level is considered the "good" cholesterol because it is responsible for removing cholesterol deposits from the arteries and carrying them to the liver for excretion. The HDL-cholesterol test is also drawn to monitor patients on lipid-lowering treatments to see if their risk for heart disease has improved.

Indications: The HDL-cholesterol is generally checked on healthy individuals every 4-6 years during a routine checkup. Patients will need lipid profile testing at an increased frequency if they have a higher risk for heart disease. It should be done more frequently in patients who have cardiovascular risk factors, such as tobacco abuse, obesity, poor dietary habits, a sedentary lifestyle, hypertension, a positive family history of heart disease, older age, preexisting heart disease, or diabetes.

Normal Range: The most desirable level for the HDL-cholesterol is any number greater than or equal to 60 mg/dL.

Critical Range: There is no critical range for the HDL-cholesterol but people with an HDL-C level of less than or equal to 40 mg/dL are considered high risk for heart disease.

Increased Value May Indicate: Increased levels of HDL-cholesterol are desirable and indicate a decreased risk for heart disease. Ideally, the HDL-C level should be at least 60 mg/dL aa this is considered a negative risk factor for heart disease.

Decreased Value May Indicate: HDL-C levels of less than 40 mg/dL in men and less than 50 mg/dL in women increase the risk for heart disease regardless of any other risk factors. The average person with an average risk for heart disease has an HDL-cholesterol level of between 40 and 50 mg/dL for men and between 50 and 59 mg/dL for women.

Factors, Risks, or Other Information: The HDL-cholesterol level shouldn't be measured when a person is acutely ill as this can temporarily lower their HDL-cholesterol. People under stress, who've had trauma, or who've had a heart attack are poor candidates to have an HDL-cholesterol drawn as it will not accurately reflect their cholesterol level when they are well. In the same way, cholesterol levels are altered in pregnancy and don't reflect an added risk for heart disease. HDL-testing should wait until after the pregnancy has passed for at least six weeks.

Triglycerides

Abbreviation: TG

How Is It Measured: The triglyceride test is part of the lipid profile drawn on fasting patients from a sampling of venous blood. The blood is stored in a red top, red/gold top, or gold top tube and is centrifuged until the serum is separated from the blood components. The serum is then electronically tested for the triglyceride level.

Description: The blood test for triglyceride level is part of a lipid profile designed to identify the risk for cardiovascular disease in healthy individuals and to make decisions as to whether or not lipid lowering treatment is to be recommended. Patients with preexisting heart disease or other risk factors also have triglyceride testing and the triglyceride level does seem to increase the risk for heart disease, independent of other risk factors.

Indications: The triglyceride level is generally checked on healthy individuals every 4-6 years during a routine checkup. Patients will need lipid profile testing, including a triglyceride level, at an increased frequency if they have a higher risk for heart disease. It should be done more frequently in patients who have cardiovascular risk factors, such as tobacco abuse, obesity, poor dietary habits, a sedentary lifestyle, hypertension, a positive family history of heart disease, older age, preexisting heart disease, or diabetes. Triglyceride testing is also done to monitor patients on a lipid-lowering program of diet, exercise, and medications in order to monitor the effectiveness of the program.

Normal Range: The desirable range for total triglyceride levels should be less than 150 mg/dL.

Desirable: Desirable: <150 mg/dL

Borderline High: 150-199 mg/dL

High Risk: 200-499 mg/dL

Very High: ≥500 mg/dL

Critical Range: There is no critical range for triglyceride testing. Instead, patients are stratified according to their triglyceride level. Patients with a triglyceride level of 150-199 mg/dL have a borderline high risk for heart disease; patients with a triglyceride level of 200-499 mg/dL have a high risk for heart disease; and patients with a triglyceride level of more than 500 mg/dL have a very high risk for heart disease. Patients with extremely high triglyceride levels in the range of 1000 mg/dL have an increased risk for pancreatitis.

Increased Value May Indicate: Patients with elevated triglyceride levels have an increased risk for both heart disease and pancreatitis, independent of other risk factors for these diseases.

Decreased Value May Indicate: There is no danger to having a low triglyceride level so that, if a low triglyceride level is found, it is not felt to be clinically significant.

Factors, Risks, or Other Information: Patients with uncontrolled diabetes tend to have very high triglyceride levels. Because the triglyceride level is extremely dependent upon diet, it must be done on a fasting basis or the test will be completely inaccurate. Certain medications, such as protease inhibitors, corticosteroids, estrogens, and beta blockers will increase the triglyceride level.

4.06 Antibody Screening

The panel of lab values consists of:

- Rheumatoid Factor

- Fluorescent Antinuclear Antibody

- Direct Coomb's Antibody Test

- Indirect Coomb's Antibody Test

- Thyroid Antibody Testing

- Human Immunodeficiency Antibody Test

Rheumatoid Factor

Abbreviation: RF or RAF

How Is It Measured: The Rheumatoid factor is a serology test done on a red top, red/gold top, or gold top tube and is obtained from venous blood in a peripheral smear. Titers are obtained at serial dilutions to find a dilution level that corresponds with a positive antibody test. This dilution is reported and higher dilution levels mean a more positive test.

Description: The rheumatoid factor or RF test is mainly a test to help in the diagnosis of rheumatoid arthritis, which is an autoimmune form of arthritis, affecting small and large joints. Rheumatoid arthritis depends on the clinical evaluation and x-rays but a RF can help clinch the diagnosis. In addition, some patients have an incomplete clinical picture and need an RF titer to help make the diagnosis. Patients can have a positive RA factor and may have another connective disease that will confuse the testing.

Indications: The RF test can be ordered for signs and symptoms of rheumatoid arthritis, including morning stiffness, joint pain, swelling and warmth of the skin, and nodules under the skin. Progressive disease will show x-ray changes and swollen joint capsules. The RF test may not be positive initially but will be positive after serial testing. The RF test is often done along with other autoimmune tests, such as the C-reactive protein, the ANA titer, and the erythrocyte sedimentation rate, which is a measure of inflammation.

Normal Range: A normal test is negative or a very low titer of less than 1:16.

Critical Range: There really isn't a critical range for this type of test as people make antibodies at different rates. Patients who are immunocompromised will have a decreased ability to make antibodies and will not have as high a titer as patients with a normal immune system. Titers may be reported as a physical number, such as 1:320, which is critically high and indicates a high titer and a positive test.

Increased Value May Indicate: The patient with signs and symptoms of rheumatoid arthritis will likely have symptoms and a high RF antibody titer. The higher the titer, the more severe is the disease. A negative test doesn't rule out rheumatoid arthritis and about twenty percent of RA patients will have a low level or negative titer. In such cases, a Cyclic Citrullinated Peptide Antibody test may need to be performed to confirm the disease. Positive RF antibody testing will be seen in 1-5 percent of normal individuals and in individuals with other connective tissue diseases. Once positive, the RF titer is not used to monitor the course of the disease.

Decreased Value May Indicate: A negative RF test does not rule out rheumatoid arthritis but should be serially tested to make sure the test turns positive at some point in the disorder.

Factors, Risks, or Other Information: According the American College of Rheumatology, both a cyclic citrullinated peptide or CPP antibody test should be done as part of an antibody screen for rheumatoid arthritis as it can be positive when the RF is negative. About 50-60 percent of people with early RA will have a positive CPP antibody test but will have a negative RF test.

Fluorescent Antinuclear Antibody

Abbreviation: FANA or ANA

How Is It Measured: The FANA or ANA is a serology test done on a red top, red/gold top, or gold top tube and is obtained from venous blood in a peripheral smear. Titers are obtained at serial dilutions to find a dilution level that corresponds with a positive antibody test. This dilution is reported and higher dilution levels mean a more positive test.

Description: The FANA or ANA test is used to identify the various autoimmune disorders that can affect the various tissues and organs of the body. It is the most common test used to diagnose systemic lupus erythematosus or SLE. ANA are actually a collection of autoantibodies produced by the immune system as antibodies unable to distinguish between foreign antibodies and self-antibodies. The target for the antibodies is the nucleus of the cell, which causes organ destruction and tissue loss. The ANA test can be done when the signs and symptoms the patient is exhibiting is indicative of a connective tissue disease of autoimmune origins. It is followed up by specific antibody tests for various autoimmune diseases, of which there are hundreds of different disorders. The ANA is reported as being "diffuse" when there is diffuse uptake of fluorescent-tagged antibodies and "speckled" when there is a non-diffuse uptake of fluorescent-tagged antibodies. The test is reported as positive or negative, or as a titer.

Indications: The ANA test is ordered when there are clinical signs and symptoms typical of a systemic autoimmune disorder. The symptoms vary according to the disorder but many patients have systemic symptoms including a low-grade fever, weakness, tiredness, arthritic joint pain, alopecia, light sensitivity, rashes, muscular soreness, paresthesias, and areas of inflamed tissues in the body.

Normal Range: The normal range is a negative test or a titer that is less than 1:8 or 1:16.

Critical Range: There really isn't a critical range for this type of test as people make antibodies at different rates. Patients who are immunocompromised will have a decreased ability to make antibodies and will not have as high a titer as patients with a normal immune system. Titers may be reported as a physical number, such as 1:320, which is critically high and indicates a high titer and a positive test.

Increased Value May Indicate: A positive ANA test means that there are autoantibodies present in the patient's body and is suggestive of autoimmune disease. The test is further done by determining the number of antibodies seen. This can be and enzyme linked immunosorbent assay or ELISA test, which reports the number of antibodies as an arbitrary number or the indirect fluorescent antibody test or IFA test which reports the actual titer that led to a positive result. For example, a titer of 1:320 means that the serum was diluted with 320 parts of a diluting solution with detectable antibodies present. The IFA will also be reported as "diffuse", as is seen in drug-induced lupus and SLE, "speckled", as is seen in Sjogren's syndrome, polymyositis, scleroderma, mixed connective tissue disease, and polymyositis, "nucleolar", as is seen in polymyositis and scleroderma or "centromere pattern", which is seen in CREST syndrome and scleroderma.

Decreased Value May Indicate: A low titer or negative test usually means the individual does not have an autoimmune disease; however, the test may have a low titer or may be negative early in the course of these diseases.

Factors, Risks, or Other Information: ANA testing is used to diagnose autoimmune diseases but is not used to track these diseases after they have been diagnosed. Autoimmune hepatitis, certain infections, drugs, and primary biliary cirrhosis, and many other autoimmune diseases can be screened for with an ANA or FANA test. About 3-6 percent of normal people under the age of 65 will have a positive ANA titer, but usually at a low titer. Older individuals are more likely to have a positive ANA test, which are false-positive tests and don't indicate an autoimmune disease is taking place.

Direct Coomb's Antibody Test

Abbreviation: DAT

How Is It Measured: The direct Coomb's antibody test is a serology test done on a red top, red/gold top, or gold top tube and is obtained from venous blood in a peripheral smear. Titers are obtained at serial dilutions to find a dilution level that corresponds with a positive antibody test. This dilution is reported and higher dilution levels mean a more positive test.

Description: The direct Coomb's antibody test or DAT is used primarily in the detection of hemolytic anemia, in which RBCs are destroyed because they have been tagged with antibodies. The antibodies may be autoantibodies as part of an autoimmune disease like autoimmune-mediated hemolytic anemia, SLE, lymphoma, chronic lymphocytic anemia, infectious mononucleosis, certain drug-induced autoimmune states, and mycoplasma pneumonia.

The direct Coomb's test is used to diagnose hemolytic disease of the newborn, which is secondary to a blood incompatibility between a mother and her infant. The mother may be exposed to fetal antigens on the baby's red blood cells, producing antibodies against them. This is especially common among Rh-negative mothers and Rh-positive infants. This has been largely eradicated by the use of the Rhogam shot in pregnancy so that ABO incompatibility is now the most common reason for hemolytic disease of the newborn.

The direct Coomb's test can also be used to evaluate a possible transfusion reaction. If there are symptoms of a transfusion reaction, the DAT is done to see if there are patient antibodies directed at the transfused RBCs. If this is the case, the transfused RBCs will be destroyed and another transfusion may be necessary.

Indications: The DAT test is ordered when there is clinical suspicion of hemolytic anemia, which can be in adults or in newborns. A baby who is pale, jaundiced, short of breath, and who has peripheral edema and liver/splenic enlargement may have hemolytic disease of the newborn.

Transfusion reaction patients with hemolysis will have back pain, fever, chills, and hematuria, necessitating a DAT test to confirm immune-mediated hemolysis of RBCs.

Normal Range: A normal test will be negative for the presence of antibodies against RBCs.

Critical Range: There really isn't a critical range for this type of test as people make antibodies at different rates. Patients who are immunocompromised will have a decreased ability to make antibodies and will not have as high a titer as patients with a normal immune system. Titers may be reported as a physical number, such as 1:320, which is critically high and indicates a high titer and a positive test.

Increased Value May Indicate: A positive DAT indicates the presence of antibodies against the RBCs. The higher the titer, the more severe the disease as there is more antibody bound to the cells. Some patients, however, can have mild symptoms and high titers, or vice versa. The positive DAT is indicative of immune-mediated hemolysis but it doesn't indicate the cause of the disease so the test must be further evaluated with a history, physical examination, and further laboratory evaluation.

Decreased Value May Indicate: A negative DAT usually means that antibodies are not attached to the RBCs and the cause of the hemolysis or transfusion reaction is not immune-mediated.

Factors, Risks, or Other Information: If the DAT is positive in a transfusion reaction, a drug reaction, or an infectious process, it can remain high as long as three months after the illness. DAT levels high for longer than that should prompt a test for an autoimmune disease.

Indirect Coomb's Antibody Test

Abbreviation: IAT

How Is It Measured: The Indirect Coomb's Antibody Test is a serology test done on a red top, red/gold top, or gold top tube and is obtained from venous blood in a peripheral smear. Titers are obtained at serial dilutions to find a dilution level that corresponds with a positive antibody test. This dilution is reported and higher dilution levels mean a more positive test.

Description: The indirect Coomb's test or IAT is and RBC antibody screen used in the screening of a person's blood for antibodies directed at the non-A and non-B antibodies on RBCs. It is used to type and screen blood prior to a transfusion or part of testing of pregnant women who might have RBC antibodies. Exposure to RBC antibodies come from prior pregnancies, prior blood transfusions, or other blood exposure to another person's blood. These can cause a severe transfusion reaction if the transfused blood is given that has the right antibodies attached to them. A positive test is not diagnostic but indicates the need for further testing to identify the type of antibody found in the patient's body. Donor blood must be sought that doesn't result in a positive IAT test. Delayed or immediate blood transfusion reactions require a DAT test, which will prompt further testing for the exact antibody if the test is positive. The IAT is tested in pregnancy for the presence of an antibody against the Rh factor in Rh negative women. The Rh-positivity comes from a reaction to the D antigen on the fetus's RBCs.

Indications: The IAT test is done prior to any anticipated blood transfusion as well as in early in pregnancy (for evidence of anti-D antibodies in Rh-negative mothers).

Normal Range: The normal indirect Coomb's test or IAT test is negative, indicating that there are no antibodies in the patient's blood that are attached to any RBC foreign antigens.

Critical Range: There really isn't a critical range for this type of test as people make antibodies at different rates. Patients who are immunocompromised will have a decreased ability to make antibodies and will not have as high a titer as patients with a normal immune system. Titers may be reported as a physical number, such as 1:320, which is critically high and indicates a high titer and a positive test.

Increased Value May Indicate: If the IAT test is positive, it means that at least one RBC antibody is present to a foreign RBC antigen and the transfusion of the blood tested should not take place. It indicates a need for further testing to check for the exact antigen affected. Donor blood must then be found that doesn't contain the particular foreign antigen or antigens on its surface.

Decreased Value May Indicate: If an Rh-negative mother has an IAT test that is negative, she is given Rhogam, which is an immune globulin injection of the Rh antigen that can prevent antibody production. The Rhogam injection is not helpful if the indirect Coomb's test for the Rh antigen is already positive in pregnancy.

Factors, Risks, or Other Information: Any circulating RBC antibody is always going to be present in the body but may reduce to undetectable levels. Unfortunately, re-exposure to the antigen will increase antibody production and a reaction against the RBCs will still occur. The more blood transfusions a person has, the greater will the chance be that they will have a positive ITA test and will have more difficulty finding compatible blood.

Thyroid Antibody Testing

Abbreviation: TPO, TGAb, TGAb, TSHRAb, TBII

Other names: Thyroid Peroxidase Antibody Test, Thyroglobulin Antibody Test, Thyroid stimulating Hormone Receptor Antibody

How Is It Measured: Thyroid antibody testing are a series of serology tests done on a red top, red/gold top, or gold top tube and is obtained from venous blood in a peripheral smear. Titers are obtained at serial dilutions to find a dilution level that corresponds with a positive antibody test. This dilution is reported and higher dilution levels mean a more positive test.

Description: The thyroid antibody testing panel includes testing for thyroid peroxidase antibody or TPO, which is a test for autoimmune thyroiditis. The antibodies are directed at thyroid cells, leading to thyroid dysfunction and a diagnosis of Hashimoto's thyroiditis. The anti-TPO antibody can be positive in Grave's disease as well. The thyroglobulin antibody or TGAb test is an antibody test for antibodies against thyroglobulin, which is the storage protein of thyroid hormones. A TSHRAb or thyroid stimulating hormone receptor antibody includes antibodies against TSH receptors, increasing thyroid function as is seen in Grave's disease. A thyroid inhibitory immunoglobulin antibody test or TBII test is a test that blocks TSH from binding to normal thyroid tissue, leading to a hypothyroid state. The TBII test is rarely used.

Indications: Thyroid antibody testing is done to evaluate a patient with a goiter or who has clinical evidence for having hypothyroidism or hyperthyroidism. When the thyroid profile is indicative of thyroid disease, a thyroid antibody panel is ordered. These will indicate the presence of an autoimmune thyroid disease but can be positive in other autoimmune diseases. Patients with thyroid cancer will specifically have an anti-thyroglobulin test to see if they have anti-thyroglobulin antibodies that might affect the level of thyroglobulin in their body. Low levels of thyroid hormones or hypothyroidism can reveal itself as tiredness, weight gain, constipation, alopecia, cold intolerance, and dry skin. Elevated levels of thyroid hormone can reveal itself as excessive sweating, anxiety, tachycardia, bulging eyes, weight loss, insomnia, fatigue, and tremors.

Normal Range: A normal level of thyroid antibodies of any sort is negative or an extremely low titer.

Critical Range: There really isn't a critical range for this type of test as people make antibodies at different rates. Patients who are immunocompromised will have a decreased ability to make antibodies and will not have as high a titer as patients with a normal immune system. Titers may be reported as a physical number, such as 1:320, which is critically high and indicates a high titer and a positive test.

Increased Value May Indicate: Increased titers of autoantibodies against thyroid diseases include having a positive thyroid peroxidase antibody in Grave's disease or Hashimoto thyroiditis. These patients are hypothyroid clinically. An antithyroglobulin antibody test will be positive in Hashimoto thyroiditis and thyroid cancer, while a positive thyroid stimulating hormone receptor antibody test and thyroid stimulating immunoglobulin test will be positive in Grave's disease and will show up as clinical hyperthyroidism.

Mildly elevated or moderately elevated anti-thyroid antibodies can be seen in other autoimmune diseases, such as type I diabetes, pernicious anemia, thyroid cancer, and autoimmune collagen vascular diseases. Very high titers are primarily seen in Hashimoto thyroiditis and Graves' disease. The higher the titer, the more severe the disease is. Pregnant women with high titers of anti-thyroid antibodies may lead to thyroid disorders in the newborn. A small percentage of patients who are normal will have positive anti-thyroid antibodies but no evidence of thyroid disease. It may indicate future autoimmune thyroid diseases.

Decreased Value May Indicate: Negative anti-thyroid antibodies with patients who have symptoms of hyperthyroidism or hypothyroidism mean the symptoms are not autoimmune-related or that the autoimmune disease is too early to have detectable autoantibodies.

Factors, Risks, or Other Information: The sensitivity and specificity of the various anti-thyroid antibody tests have improved over time but still are not perfect. There are several different anti-thyroid antibodies that can be tested for and that can be matched with clinical symptoms to make a thyroid diagnosis that is autoimmune-mediated.

Human Immunodeficiency Antibody Test

Abbreviation: HIV Screening

Other names: Human Immunodeficiency Antigen Test

How Is It Measured: HIV antibody screening is a serology test done on a red top, red/gold top, or gold top tube and is obtained from venous blood in a peripheral smear. Titers are obtained at serial dilutions to find a dilution level that corresponds with a positive antibody test. This dilution is reported and higher dilution levels mean a more positive test. The human immunodeficiency antigen test is either a positive or negative test.

Description: HIV antibody testing and HIV antibody testing (p24 testing) are used together to screen for the presence of HIV infections. It is crucial to detect this disorder as quickly as possible as antiretroviral medications are available that can slow the progression of the disease and can improve survival rates. Screening testing can be done by testing for the HIV antigen and HIV antibody together. Both HIV-1 and HIV-2 are tested for. HIV-1 has a higher prevalence in the US, while HIV-2 has a higher prevalence in Africa. The p24 antigen test and the viral load test are high right after an acute infection so these can be done to detect early disease before antibodies have been made. Antibodies can be present within two weeks of exposure but the combination of antibody and antigen testing is the preferred way to screen for the disorder. These are just screening tests and must be followed by confirmatory testing for a different HIV antibody. RNA material for the HIV test can be a confirmatory test as can an HIV0RNA test, which will be positive 1-4 weeks after the infection.

Indications: The test is indicated for patients at high risk for HIV disease and pregnant women without any symptoms. All sexually-active young people should be screened if they live in areas where HIV is prevalent. Annual screening is recommended for individuals who have had unprotected sex that is not monogamous, homosexual men, illicit drug users, prostitutes, those with an HIV-positive sexual partner, and any patient with other STDs, tuberculosis, hepatitis B, or hepatitis C. Healthcare workers should be tested upon exposure to blood or body fluids.

Normal Range: A normal range for an HIV antibody test is negative and a normal range for an HIV antigen test is negative.

Critical Range: There really isn't a critical range for this type of test as people make antibodies at different rates. Patients who are immunocompromised will have a decreased ability to make antibodies and will not have as high a titer as patients with a normal immune system. Titers may be reported as a physical number, such as 1:320, which is critically high and indicates a high titer and a positive test. Any positive antigen test for the HIV antigen is considered critical.

Increased Value May Indicate: HIV testing for the antibody will not detect the antibody initially but will show detectable antibody levels 3-12 weeks after exposure. This means that repeat testing must be done on negative patients at high risk for the disease. The HIV antibody/HIV antigen test should be done on high risk patients as early as possible after exposure. A positive HIV test will prompt a test to see the type of HIV the patient has an HIV-2 RNA test if this is negative, confirming the diagnosis of an HIV-1 infection, even if anti-HIV-1 test is negative.

Decreased Value May Indicate: A negative HIV antigen and a negative HIV antibody test usually means that the patient has no HIV disease. High risk patients must always be tested serially for up to three months after exposure to make sure there isn't a late positive test. Even negatively tested patients should have an annual screening test.

Factors, Risks, or Other Information: There is no cure for an HIV infection but early detection allows for the early starting of antiretroviral therapy that will decrease the viral load and prolong survival. Several antiretroviral agents are given to target various parts of the HIV virus. There is no available vaccine for the HIV virus so avoiding exposure is the only way to prevent the disease at present. Pre-exposure prophylaxis or PEP is advised for very high risk patients to avoid getting the infection. Pregnant mothers are tested for HIV because they can take antiretroviral therapy in pregnancy, thus decreasing the chance of passing the infection on to the infant. Patients born to HIV positive mothers will receive antiretroviral therapy upon birth for six weeks to decrease the transmission rate from up to a third to less than 2 percent.

4.07 Iron Panel

The panel of lab values consists of:

- Serum Iron Level
- Total Iron Binding Capacity
- Ferritin

Serum Iron Level

Abbreviation: Fe

How Is It Measured: The serum iron level is a serum test that is drawn from a venipuncture and is used from blood placed in a red top tube, a red/gold top tube, or a gold top tube from which serum is collected after centrifuging whole blood to separate the serum from the blood products. The serum iron level is then electronically determined.

Description: A patient's iron status actually is determined by several tests, each of which will be discussed separately. The serum iron test is a measure of the iron in serum and is a test that can help identify states of elevated serum iron or states of low serum iron. While the serum iron test is important, it can rarely diagnose an iron-related disease unless it is checked with some of the other iron studies.

Indications: A serum iron test is often done when a CBC shows a low hematocrit, indicating iron-deficiency anemia. These patients will have chronic fatigue, pale skin, weakness, and dizziness from a lack of iron and oxygen-carrying capacity. Cases of suspected iron overload can be measured with a serum iron level. Patients suspected of this disorder will have heart abnormalities, low libido, abdominal discomfort, lack of energy, fatigue, muscle weakness, and pain in the joints.

Normal Range: Men have higher serum iron levels than women in the range of about 65-176 micrograms per deciliter. Adult women will have normal iron levels of between 50 and 270 micrograms per deciliter. The iron is generally bound to transferrin when measured as up to a third of all body transferrin will contain iron.

Critical Range: There are no critical values for the serum iron level. If the patient has iron toxicity and needs chelation therapy, the serum total ferritin level is assessed to see if the chelation is working.

Increased Value May Indicate: Elevated serum iron levels will be seen in hemochromatosis, which is a hereditary iron overload disease. There will be a high transferrin saturation and a high ferritin level. Hemolytic anemia patients and patients will have high serum iron levels and both high percent saturation of transferrin and high ferritin levels. Children or adults with iron ingestion, will have a high iron level, a high percent transferrin saturation level, but will have normal ferritin levels. Patients with hereditary hemochromatosis may have no symptoms but will have a markedly elevated serum iron level. As they age, symptoms of joint pain, abdominal discomfort, and weakness may develop, starting at age 30 years. Patients who had multiple transfusions will have high serum iron levels because the iron from transfused blood will remain in the body and build up in the person's tissues.

Decreased Value May Indicate: Decreased serum iron will be seen in hemochromatosis with low iron stores and low percent transferrin saturation levels. Patients with chronic diseases will have low iron levels in the blood, low transferrin saturation levels, and normal or high ferritin levels. Mild cases of iron deficiency will only have low ferritin stores but will have a normal serum iron level. As the iron deficiency worsens, the iron stores will be depleted and the serum iron will drop. The TIBC (Total Iron Binding Capacity) will increase as the protein levels will rise to collect as much iron as possible.

Factors, Risks, or Other Information: Normal serum iron levels happen by a regulation of the intake of iron and slow but gradual loss of iron daily by the body. If the dietary intake is low, iron deficiency anemia will result. If there are excess iron losses from occult or obvious bleeding, iron deficiency anemia will result. Pregnant women are prone to low serum iron levels as they need an increased iron intake during the pregnancy. Chronic diseases, such as autoimmune disease, AIDS, and cancers have low iron because they cannot use iron in their body and will have both low serum transferrin levels and low iron levels with the iron just being stored as ferritin.

Total Iron Binding Capacity

Abbreviation: TIBC

How Is It Measured: The total iron binding capacity is a serum test that is drawn from a venipuncture and is used from blood placed in a red top tube, a red/gold top tube, or a gold top tube from which serum is collected after centrifuging whole blood to separate the serum from the blood products. The serum iron binding capacity is then electronically determined.

Description: The TIBC is often done alongside a serum iron level to see what type of iron disorder the patient has. The TIBC and the serum iron together are used to calculate the percent of transferrin saturation, which is a useful indicator of the person's true iron status. About 20-40 percent of the available transferrin is used to transport iron in the bloodstream. Iron deficiency anemia, the most common type of iron disorder will have a high TIBC but a low transferrin saturation level because there is little iron in the body. In hemochromatosis, both the serum iron and TIBC will be low or normal, resulting in an increase in transferrin to carry the excess iron. Transferrin levels are low in liver disease as this protein is made by the liver.

Indications: The TIBC and serum iron are ordered together when iron deficiency or iron overload are suspected. A total CBC may be performed to assess the outcome of the iron levels and TIBC levels in the blood. Symptoms of anemia include fatigue, muscle weakness, dizziness, pale skin, and headaches. Iron overload or hemochromatosis are evaluated with a serum iron and TIBC. They build up as the iron level increases, leading to tiredness, joint pain, abdominal discomfort, weight loss, low energy levels, low libido, and alopecia. Many patients are, however, asymptomatic.

Normal Range: As mentioned, the TIBC is often done along with the serum iron level. The measurement is that of the total iron binding capacity of transferrin molecules available to bind to serum. The range for transferrin is 240-400 micrograms/dL, with a percent transferrin saturation of between 11 and 46 percent.

Critical Range: There are no critical ranges available for the TIBC, although it can be markedly high in severe iron deficiency anemia and markedly low in hemochromatosis.

Increased Value May Indicate: TIBC levels indicate the amount of transferrin in the body available to bind iron. It is elevated in iron deficiency anemia, when the body attempts to correct itself by having as much transferrin available for the binding of iron.

Decreased Value May Indicate: Low TIBC levels are seen in patients with hemochromatosis, anemias with elevated iron levels, malnutrition, inflammation, nephrotic syndrome, other kidney diseases, and liver disease with low protein level production. The percent transferrin saturation is decreased in iron deficiency states and increased in iron overload or iron poisoning.

Factors, Risks, or Other Information: Having a recent blood transfusion can throw off the serum iron results as patients with clinical iron deficiency anemia may have iron overload with normal TIBC levels as the body has not had time to compensate by building serum transferrin proteins.

Ferritin

Abbreviation: Ferr

How Is It Measured: The total body ferritin level is an estimated serum test that is drawn from a venipuncture and is used from blood placed in a red top tube, a red/gold top tube, or a gold top tube from which serum is collected after centrifuging whole blood to separate the serum from the blood products. The serum is then electronically determined and approximates the total body ferritin level.

Description: The serum ferritin level is a test done to measure the iron stores in the body. The test is ordered along with the TIBC and serum iron level to best understand the patient's iron disorder.

Indications: The main indications for the test is to evaluate the meaning behind abnormalities of the CBC, such as a low hemoglobin level or a high hematocrit level. In the early stages of iron deficiency anemia, the patient will have a mildly low hemoglobin, low ferritin stores, and very few symptoms. As the ferritin levels drop and iron stores diminish, the patient has symptoms of iron deficiency anemia, including weakness, chronic fatigue, headaches, dizziness, pale skin, and shortness of breath. As the iron stores become depleted, the anemia worsens, and things like shock and heart failure can occur. Children will have cognitive deficits, and some patients will exhibit pica and some will have spoon-shaped nails. The ferritin level may also be ordered when a patient is suspected to have hemochromatosis or other iron overload syndrome.

Normal Range: The normal serum ferritin is between 15 and 200 ng/ml for women 20 and 300 ng/ml for men. About 95 percent of people will have normal serum ferritin levels.

Critical Range: The optimal serum ferritin level is 25-75 ng/ml so ferritin levels higher than this, particularly above 300 ng/ml will increase the risk for liver disease, stroke, diabetes, cancer, and heart disease.

Increased Value May Indicate: High ferritin levels are interpreted best by also checking the TIBC and serum iron levels. High ferritin levels are primarily seen in iron overload states, such as hemochromatosis but can be elevated in patients with chronic disease, hemolytic anemia, and sideroblastic anemia. Because ferritin is an acute phase reactant protein, it can be high in acute inflammation, chronic infections, autoimmune disorders, liver disease, and certain cancers.

Decreased Value May Indicate: Low serum ferritin levels are mainly seen in patients with iron deficiency anemia because they have an overall low level or stored iron.

Factors, Risks, or Other Information: The bulk of ferritin is intracellular with only a small amount in the bloodstream. Damage to organs that store ferritin, such as the bone marrow, spleen, and liver, will elevate serum ferritin levels even though there is no change in the total body stores of iron and the serum ferritin level will be spuriously high.

4.08 Kidney Function Tests

The serum BUN (blood urea nitrogen) and Cr (creatinine) have already been covered as they are usually ordered as part of the serum basic metabolic panel and are not generally ordered as isolated kidney function tests, although this can certainly be done if they are ordered separately.

The panel of lab values consists of:

- Glomerular Filtration Rate
- Blood Urea Nitrogen
- Creatinine

Glomerular Filtration Rate

Abbreviation: GFR or eGFR

How Is It Measured: The GFR or glomerular filtration rate is a totally calculated number based on the patient's age and blood creatinine level. The creatinine is drawn from venous blood in a peripheral vein and collected into a red, red/gold/or gold top tube. The serum is separated from the blood components and the creatinine level is determined electronically.

Description: The test most people have is an estimated GFR, which is a screening test for early kidney disease and is helpful in diagnosing chronic kidney disease. It should be calculated every time the serum creatinine is drawn. Both the creatinine and eGFR are used to monitor patients with progressive kidney failure to see who need dialysis and when. Patients with hypertension and diabetes also have an eGFR measured during routine checkups at least every year.

Indications: The main indications for evaluating an eGFR on a patient would be to monitor their kidney function over time. Signs and symptoms that might prompt an eGFR investigation include having peripheral edema, urinary changes, oliguria, flank pain, or nocturia. Severe kidney disease has even more prominent symptoms, including polyuria, pruritus, fatigue, poor appetite, increased skin pigmentation, paresthesias, and muscle cramps. This is an excellent test for the primary monitoring of chronic renal failure.

Normal Range: A normal range for the GFR is 90-120 ml/min/1.73m^2.

Critical Range: A critical GFR is anything less than 20 ml/min/1.73m^2, which indicates the need for dialysis.

Increased Value May Indicate: There is no clinical significance associated with a high eGFR rate.

Decreased Value May Indicate: The eGFR is measured in ml/min/1.73m^2. Because some laboratories don't collect information on race so the eGFR is reported for both Caucasians and African Americans. The number is calculated until the level is less than 60 ml/min/1.73 m^2. Any eGFR below 60 ml/min/1.73m^2 suggests kidney damage and should be followed routinely. The eGFR is not the only way to predict kidney damage so things like a urine albumin level may need to be obtained.

Factors, Risks, or Other Information: There is another way to evaluate the GFR is to measure the cystatin C level. This test is superior to using the creatinine level and may be a test and evaluation measurement for the eGFR in the future. The creatinine clearance test can also measure the GFR accurately and directly but requires a precise 24-hour urine collection in order to obtain the necessary lab parameters to calculate the GFR. The GFR naturally decreases with age and naturally increases in pregnancy.

4.09 Liver Function Testing

The panel of lab values consists of:

- Aspartate Aminotransferase
- Alanine Aminotransferase
- Total Bilirubin
- Serum Ammonia Level

Aspartate Aminotransferase

Abbreviation: AST

How Is It Measured: The AST level is a serum test that is drawn from a venipuncture and is used from blood placed in a red top tube, a red/gold top tube, or a gold top tube from which serum is collected after centrifuging whole blood to separate the serum from the blood products. The AST level is then electronically determined.

Description: The serum AST or aspartate aminotransferase is usually drawn to detect liver damage. It is often ordered with the ALT or alanine aminotransferase as part of a liver panel or sometimes as part of a comprehensive metabolic panel or CMP. It is used to diagnose liver disorders. The AST is one of the most important test for evaluation of liver function because it is directly produced from hepatocytes. The ratio of AST and ALT are important in distinguishing the type of liver disorder the patient has. The AST is not as specific for liver damage as is the ALT. The AST can be drawn as an individual test for the monitoring of potential liver problems in the taking of hepatotoxic medications.

Indications: The major indications for an AST test is for routine screening of healthy patients as part of routine health screening. The

AST can also be drawn when there is a suspicious clinical picture for liver disease, including anorexia, tiredness, nausea, vomiting, ascites, jaundice, dark urine, pruritus, peripheral edema, and easy bruisability. AST levels are also drawn with patient who have no evidence of liver disease but have been exposed to the hepatitis virus, drink heavily, have a history of familial liver disease, are taking hepatotoxic drugs, or patients with diabetes.

Normal Range: The normal range for AST varies according to the laboratory but is about 10-40 units per liter.

Critical Range: There is no critical level for the AST. Elevated levels can be up to 100 times normal in liver toxicity situations, indicating severe liver disease.

Increased Value May Indicate: Extremely high AST levels of at least ten times the normal range are suspicious for acute viral hepatitis. These levels can last for up to six months before resolving. AST levels can be a hundred times normal when a patient has taken a hepatotoxic drug or is suffering from liver ischemia.

With chronic hepatitis, the AST levels are minimally high, up to four times normal and tend to remain elevated longer than the ALT level. Cirrhosis of the liver will also have slightly elevated AST levels. Muscle injury and heart attacks will raise AST levels from non-hepatic sources. In most cases of liver disease, the ALT level is elevated to a greater degree than the AST unless the source is the heart or muscle injury.

Decreased Value May Indicate: There are no clinical conditions associated with a low AST so this is considered a normal finding.

Factors, Risks, or Other Information: Women who are pregnant, those receiving IM injections, and patients who strenuously exercise may have an increase in AST levels. Surgery, seizures and major burns will elevate the AST level. Certain drugs and herbal preparations can inflame the liver, resulting in AST elevations.

Alanine Aminotransferase

Abbreviation: ALT

How Is It Measured: The ALT level is a serum test that is drawn from a venipuncture and is used from blood placed in a red top tube, a red/gold top tube, or a gold top tube from which serum is collected after centrifuging whole blood to separate the serum from the blood products. The ALT level is then electronically determined.

Description: The ALT or alanine aminotransferase level is used to check for liver injury. It is often used in conjunction with the AST test as part of a liver panel used to diagnose screen for liver disease. ALT is produced primarily by the hepatocytes and renal cells. When there is liver damage, the ALT will be elevated, making it a good marker for any type of liver disease. As the AST level can be elevated in non-liver conditions, the ALT is considered more specific to liver injury. The AST/ALT ratio is always calculated to detect liver versus non-liver injuries. The total protein, alkaline phosphatase, and total bilirubin are sometimes assessed to see what liver disorder might be present.

Indications: The major indications for an ALT test is for routine screening of healthy patients as part of routine health screening. The ALT can also be drawn when there is a suspicious clinical picture for liver disease, including anorexia, tiredness, nausea, vomiting, ascites, jaundice, dark urine, pruritus, peripheral edema, and easy bruisability. ALT levels are also drawn with patient who have no evidence of liver disease but have been exposed to the hepatitis virus, drink heavily, have a history of familial liver disease, are taking hepatotoxic drugs, or patients with diabetes. The ALT test is more specific to liver disease than the AST so liver disease should be suspected if this test is elevated.

Normal Range: The normal level of ALT will vary slightly from laboratory to laboratory but is usually about 7-56 units per liter.

Critical Range: There is no critical range for the ALT level but it can be a much as 100 times normal or more in severe liver failure or when taking hepatoxic drugs.

Increased Value May Indicate: Levels of ALT greater than ten times normal can be seen in acute hepatitis, which is usually viral. The ALT levels may take up to six months to normalize after viral hepatitis. Levels more than 100 times normal are seen in acute liver failure or liver toxicity from hepatotoxic drugs. ALT levels are not usually high in chronic hepatitis but can be up to four times the normal range. Moderate increases in ALT can be seen in liver cirrhosis, heart damage, metastatic liver disease, and bile duct obstruction. Expect the ALT to be higher in liver-related diseases, with an ALT to AST ratio of greater than one in things like acute hepatitis, alcoholic hepatitis, liver cirrhosis, heart muscle damage, or muscle injury.

Decreased Value May Indicate: Low ALT levels in the blood are to be expected and are not related to any particular liver disease.

Factors, Risks, or Other Information: Intramuscular injections and strenuous activity will increase the ALT levels. Certain drugs will cause liver damage in high-risk patient and certain herbs will raise the ALT due to liver cell damage.

Total Bilirubin

Abbreviation: TBili, Indirect Bili, Direct Bili

Other Names: Indirect Bilirubin, Direct Bilirubin

How Is It Measured: The bilirubin is a serum test that is drawn from a venipuncture and is used from blood placed in a red top tube, a red/gold top tube, or a gold top tube from which serum is collected after centrifuging whole blood to separate the serum from the blood products. The bilirubin level is then electronically determined. In neonates, the indirect bilirubin is assessed by doing a heel stick and obtaining about one milliliter of blood.

Description: A bilirubin test is used to detect the release of bilirubin or buildup of bilirubin from the breakdown of heme. Bilirubin elevations cause jaundice and can be seen in hemolytic anemia or liver disease. Bile duct blockage will prevent bilirubin processing and will raise the bilirubin. There are two forms of bilirubin measured by the lab. The first is the unconjugated or indirect bilirubin. This is the bilirubin directly released from heme but is not yet processed by the liver. The second is conjugated bilirubin, formed after the liver attaches sugar to the bilirubin. This is the bilirubin found in the bile and that which is passed through the stool. Generally, the total bilirubin is assessed and, if this is abnormal, the direct or "water soluble" bilirubin is obtained. The indirect bilirubin is then calculated from these two levels.

Indications: In adults and older children, the bilirubin is evaluated to monitor and diagnose diseases of the liver and its bile ducts. Patients with hemolytic anemia or sickle cell anemia will have elevations of the total bilirubin from an increase in unconjugated bilirubin. In newborns, the unconjugated bilirubin is evaluated to check for physiological or pathological causes of jaundice. It is rare to have elevations in bilirubin in newborns because of newborn hepatitis or biliary atresia. These will increase the direct bilirubin as well as the indirect bilirubin. The bilirubin is checked along with liver enzymes when jaundice is detected, when there is clinical evidence of excessive alcohol use or drug toxicity, or when there has been an exposure to a hepatitis virus.

Normal Range: The normal range for total bilirubin level in adults is 0.0 to 1.4 mg/dL. The normal range for the direct hemoglobin 0.0-0.3 mg/dL. The normal range for indirect bilirubin Is 0.2-1.2 mg/dL

Critical Range: There is no critical lab value for bilirubin. The bilirubin can be 0.0 mg/dL and this can be normal. Jaundice is present when the bilirubin level reaches about 10 mg/dL but the level can go higher than that. An indirect bilirubin of about 17 mg/dL or more in neonates is considered pathologic and warrants immediate intervention.

Increased Value May Indicate: In adults and children, high levels of total bilirubin can indicate hemolytic anemia, transfusion reaction, Gilbert syndrome, or cirrhosis if the bilirubin is mostly unconjugated. Elevations in conjugated bilirubin are more common and is usually seen in liver injuries such as alcoholic liver disease, drug reactions, or viral hepatitis. Blockage of the bile ducts will elevate the direct bilirubin level. This can happen from fibrosis of the bile ducts, gallstones, or tumors of the bile ducts. Physiologic jaundice with unconjugated bilirubin levels of up to 12 mg/dL are physiologic. Higher levels may be pathological and may be caused by an accelerated loss of RBCs as can be seen with hemolytic anemia from ABO incompatibility with the mother's blood, congenital infectious diseases, or acute hypoxia. Rarely, liver disease can cause indirect bilirubin elevations in neonates. Direct bilirubin elevations in neonates almost always means biliary atresia or neonatal hepatitis.

Decreased Value May Indicate: There are no clinical conditions associated with a low bilirubin level.

Factors, Risks, or Other Information: Although indirect bilirubin can be toxic to the brains of neonates up to a month of age, it does not cause the same problems in older children or in adults. The blood-brain barrier in older individuals prevents the passage of bilirubin into the brain.

Serum Ammonia Level

Abbreviation: NH3

How Is It Measured: The ammonia level is a serum test that is drawn from a venipuncture from peripheral blood and is used from blood placed in a red top tube, a red/gold top tube, or a gold top tube from which serum is collected after centrifuging whole blood to separate the serum from the blood products. The serum ammonia level is then electronically determined.

Description: The ammonia test is a direct test for the ammonia level in the blood that can be caused by severe liver dysfunction, severe kidney failure, Reye's syndrome or a genetic problem with the urea cycle. Elevated ammonia levels cause behavioral and cognitive deficits that can trigger a loss of consciousness and coma. Ammonia is a natural waste product from the digestion of bacteria in the intestines. It is usually processed by the liver but, if this doesn't happen, it can accumulate in the brain, where it becomes toxic to brain cells. The ammonia level is sometimes used to check the effectiveness of the treatment for an elevated blood ammonia level.

Indications: The ammonia test can be done on newborns with liver dysfunction, viral illnesses, or evidence of Reye syndrome if they show evidence of increased irritability, vomiting, seizures, and lethargy of unknown etiology. Most adults will have the ammonia test to evaluate symptoms related to kidney failure and liver disease. Liver function tests are ordered at the same time to evaluate the cause and severity of liver disease. Patients with liver disease that is stable can have an ammonia level drawn periodically.

Normal Range: The normal range for the serum ammonia level is 15-45 micrograms per deciliter (mcg/deciliter). (The laboratories have slightly different ranges for serum ammonia).

Critical Range: There are no critical ranges for ammonia. Any level above 45 micrograms per deciliter may cause some degree of encephalopathy and should be cause for concern.

Increased Value May Indicate: Very high ammonia levels in the serum is indicative of not appropriately processing and excreting ammonia, causing encephalopathic symptoms. In infants with an inherited urea cycle enzyme deficiency or hemolytic disease will have short-term increases in ammonia level, sometimes causing symptoms and sometimes not causing symptoms. Reye syndrome can easily be identified by having a low glucose and a high ammonia level. This can be seen in babies, children and teens. Adults usually have ammonia encephalopathy from severer liver or kidney disease.

Decreased Value May Indicate: Low ammonia levels can be seen in essential hypertension and in malignant hypertension.

Factors, Risks, or Other Information: It should be known that hepatic encephalopathy can be seen in patients who have normal ammonia levels because ammonia can build up in the brain with normal levels seen in the serum. GI bleeding with RBC hemolysis, muscular exertion, tourniquet use, and the use of certain drugs, like narcotics, valproic acid, barbiturates, diuretics, and alcohol can temporarily increase the ammonia level, as can cigarette smoking.

4.10 Lumbar Puncture

The panel of lab values consists of:

- Lumbar Puncture

Lumbar Puncture

Abbreviation: LP

How Is It Measured: A lumbar puncture is performed by having the patient placed on their side and curled up into a ball. An area between L2-L3, L3-L4, or L4-L5 is determined to be the widest and is prepped with povidone iodine. The area between the spinal processes can be given a local anesthesia. A long needle with a stylus inside is inserted until the space containing spinal fluid is obtained. The stylus is removed so that cerebrospinal fluid is allowed to drip out. In tube 1, CSF is placed into a gray top tube for evaluation of the cell count. In tube 2, glucose and protein levels are evaluated from collected CSF. In tube 3, fluid is collected for Gram stain and culture. In tube 4, CSF is collected for another cell count and differential. Only a few drops of fluid need to be obtained for each tube. The stylus is replaced, the needle is removed, and hemostasis is achieved by placing manual pressure on the puncture site for about five minutes.

Description: The lumbar puncture is actually an evaluation of several things. A Gram stain and culture of the CSF is done for an evaluation of infection, such as meningitis, cell counts and differentials can evaluate the CSF for blood, as in a subarachnoid hemorrhage. Sugar and protein levels are done to diagnose diseases like Guillain-Barre syndrome or multiple sclerosis. The pressure of the CSF is measured for increased intracranial pressure.

Indications: The main indications for a lumbar puncture is to accurately evaluate a patient for meningitis, cancer of the CSF, inflammation or bleeding near the brain, multiple sclerosis, Guillain-Barre disease, or states of increased intracerebral pressure. Contrast medium can be placed in the CSF and an x-ray can be obtained as part of an x-ray myelogram of the lumbar spine. Rarely, fluid can be removed from the spinal cord space in cases of excess spinal fluid.

Normal Range: The normal CSF pressure in adults is about 90-180 mm water. For children less than 8 years, the CSF pressure is 80-100 mm water. The normal protein level in CSF is 15-45 mg/dL with slightly higher results in children and older adults. The normal range for CSF glucose content is 40-70 mg/dL. The normal range for cell count is no red blood cells and less than 5 WBCs/mm^3. There should be no tumor cells or infectious organisms in the CSF.

Critical Range: There is no critical range for CSF levels. The sum total of all of the evaluations listed above are together interpreted to indicate spinal or CSF pathology if any of the values are not within the normal range.

Increased Value May Indicate: Higher than normal WBCs suggest an infection or leukemia in the CSF. Encephalitis, meningitis, and bacterial infections will have a high percentage of PMNs in the CSF. Protein assessment should show low levels. If these are high in the CSF, several disorders can be possible. An evaluation of the protein level can be a clue to otherwise unsuspected neurologic disease such as multiple sclerosis. The high protein levels in MS, or post-infectious states, can be informative. If the spinal tap is traumatic, protein levels can be spuriously high. The glucose level in the CSF is about sixty percent of the glucose level of the peripheral blood so that if the CSF glucose is important to evaluate, a blood glucose should be drawn at the same time. High blood glucose levels usually mean diabetes.

Decreased Value May Indicate: Low levels of white blood cells, red blood cells, and protein are normal in CSF and shouldn't indicate any pathology. Low glucose levels in the CSF could indicate bacterial meningitis but not viral meningitis. A brain hemorrhage can cause a low glucose level several days after the bleeding commences.

Factors, Risks, or Other Information: The lumbar puncture is generally safe; however, some patients may have a cerebrospinal fluid leak after the spinal tap. This involves having a headache that doesn't disappear after a couple of days. A CSF leak may be treated by doing a blood patch, which involves injecting a few milliliters of the patient's own blood is removed from vein, which clots and covers the opening made by the initial spinal tap. Headache occurs in 20-70 percent of patients who have a spinal tap. This is usually a self-limited problem that resolves within a week, even without a blood patch.

4.11 Thyroid Function Tests

The panel of lab values consists of:

- Thyroid Stimulating Hormone
- Thyroxine
- Triiodothyronine (Free T3)
- Thyroglobulin

Thyroid Stimulating Hormone

Abbreviation: TSH

How Is It Measured: The TSH level is a serum test that is drawn from a venipuncture from a peripheral vein and is used from blood placed in a red top tube, a red/gold top tube, or a gold top tube from which serum is collected after centrifuging whole blood to separate the serum from the blood products. The serum TSH level is then electronically determined.

Description: The thyroid stimulating hormone or TSH test is the best way to evaluate a person's thyroid function and to evaluate a patient for hypothyroidism or hyperthyroidism. TSH is made by the pituitary gland near the brain and is stimulated by low levels of T4 and T3 in the bloodstream. The TSH can be drawn alone or as part of a thyroid panel that includes a free T4 level, a free T3 level, and thyroid antibody studies. The main purposes of testing the TSH level is to diagnose a thyroid problem in a symptomatic patient, to screen newborns for hypothyroidism, to monitor the effectiveness of hypothyroidism therapy, to monitor the effectiveness of hyperthyroidism therapy, and sometimes to evaluate the function of the pituitary gland.

Indications: The main reason that a serum TSH is done is when someone has symptoms of hyperthyroidism or hypothyroidism or when a patient has a goiter and the physician needs to know if this represents an underactive or overactive thyroid state. Elevated thyroid function can be seen as having palpitations, weight loss, anxiety, insomnia, tremors, diarrhea, weakness, visual changes, and sometimes bulging of the eyes. If the thyroid function is low, common symptoms include constipation, dry skin, dry hair, weight gain, puffiness of the skin, cold intolerance, alopecia, tiredness, and menstrual irregularities. TSH screening is done on all newborns to evaluate for neonatal hypoglycemia.

Normal Range: The normal range for the TSH is 0.6-6.0 uU/ml.

Critical Range: There really is no critical range for the TSH level. Any levels that run outside of the normal range warrant an evaluation for hyperthyroidism (if the TSH is low) or hypothyroidism (if the TSH is high).

Increased Value May Indicate: High TSH levels mean that the patient may have an underactive thyroid gland that in not putting out enough T3 or T4, causing a feedback loop that increases the serum TSH level. Patients may simply have an underactive thyroid gland from an autoimmune state, such as Hashimoto's thyroiditis, or may have had surgical removal of the thyroid gland for cancer or an overactive thyroid state. In rare cases, an elevated TSH may indicate an adenoma of the pituitary gland producing TSH.

Decreased Value May Indicate: A low TSH may indicate hyperthyroidism or a person taking too much thyroid replacement hormone. Patients with damage to the pituitary gland will not have enough TSH and will have a low serum TSH level.

Factors, Risks, or Other Information: It is crucial to remember that the TSH level is just a quick picture of what is happening in the patient's body and may not be a representation of the total picture going on in the patient. Things that affect the TSH level include taking estrogens, having increases in the proteins that bind T4 and T3, having liver disease, being pregnant, having some type of systemic illness, or having an acquired or congenital resistance to thyroid hormones.

Thyroxine

Abbreviation: T4

How Is It Measured: The T4 or free thyroxine level is a serum test that is drawn from a venipuncture and is used from blood placed in a red top tube, a red/gold top tube, or a gold top tube from which serum is collected after centrifuging whole blood to separate the serum from the blood products. The serum free thyroxine is then electronically determined.

Description: The free T4 or free thyroxine level is used to help evaluate a patient's thyroid function in a variety of diseases of the thyroid gland. Both hypothyroidism and hyperthyroidism can be diagnosed with a free T4 level, although it is best evaluated along with a serum TSH level. The T4 level represents a measurement of one of the hormones that control the metabolism of the cells of the body. Most T4 is found bound to thyroglobulin in the body. Blood tests can measure the free T4 level or the total T4 level. The total T4 level is what is generally ordered and evaluate but it can be artificially high or low because of the level of thyroglobulin in the blood. Free T4 is not affected by the thyroglobulin levels in the body and is a more accurate picture of the person's thyroid function than the total T4 level.

Indications: A free T4 level can be ordered when an individual has signs or symptoms of hypothyroidism or hyperthyroidism and has an abnormal TSH level. Evidence of hyperthyroidism were discussed above an evidence hypothyroidism were discussed above. Patients may have severe symptoms or very mild symptoms, depending on the levels of free T4 and free T3. The free T4 test is just one test that can be done to evaluate a person with thyroid disorders.

Normal Range: The normal range for free T4 is 0.7 to 1.9 ng/dL, while the normal range for the total T4 is 4.6-12 micrograms per dL.

Critical Range: There is no critical range for the thyroxine level. Levels outside of the normal range need further evaluation with a complete thyroid profile.

Increased Value May Indicate: Increased free T4 levels usually indicate hyperthyroidism, although it is a good idea to confirm this with a TSH level, which can tell if the thyroid problem is from the pituitary gland or from the pituitary gland. The elevated free T4 level is not diagnostic of hyperthyroidism but can lead the way to further testing that will be diagnostic of the disorder.

Decreased Value May Indicate: Decreased values of free T4 usually indicate hypothyroidism but this must be confirmed by a serum TSH level. Low levels of free T4 can be due to dysfunction of the thyroid gland itself with an elevated TSH or can be due to a pituitary dysfunction, with a low TSH.

Factors, Risks, or Other Information: Generally, thyroid function testing and the T4 level should not be done in a patient who is ill or in the hospital because an acute illness can throw off the free T4 level and other thyroid function studies. Things that can affect the total T4 level include pregnancy, the taking of estrogen, liver dysfunction, acute illness, and resistance to thyroid hormones. Many of these things affect the total T4 level because it affects the protein levels in the body but don't affect the free T4 level, which is unaffected by protein levels.

Triiodothyronine

Abbreviation: Free T3

How Is It Measured: The free T3 level is a serum test that is drawn from a venipuncture and is used from blood placed in a red top tube, a red/gold top tube, or a gold top tube from which serum is collected after centrifuging whole blood to separate the serum from the blood products. The serum free T3 level is then electronically determined.

Description: The free T3 level and the total T3 levels can be assessed as part of a total blood panel that assesses the thyroid function and may be ordered to help monitor the patient with either hypothyroidism or hypothyroidism. Triiodothyronine is produced by the cells of the thyroid gland, which is responsible for cellular metabolism. The TSH level exerts a positive stimulatory effect on the production of T3, and the level of T3, when elevated, exerts a negative feedback on the TSH level, causing it to go down in the presence of high T3 levels. The total picture of the thyroid state is determined by drawing an entire thyroid panel, including the T4 level and the TSH level. Remember that most of the T3 in the body is bound to thyroglobulin so the total T3 level is affected by the thyroglobulin level but the free T3 level is not. Anti-thyroid antibodies can be drawn along with the T3 level to assess the patient for Graves' disease or Hashimoto thyroiditis.

Indications: The free T3 or total T3 level may be ordered when the screening TSH level is abnormal to assess the total picture of the patient's thyroid function. It may be ordered when hyperthyroidism is suspected and the free T4 is normal as the free T3 alone can be elevated and can result in hyperthyroid symptoms. In cases of T3 hyperthyroidism, the free T3 level is done to monitor the condition and the effectiveness of anti-thyroid drugs.

Normal Range: The normal level for the total T3 level is 80-180 ng/dL, while the normal level for the free T3 level is 230-619 pg/dL.

Critical Range: There is no particular critical range for the free T3 or total T3 level. Any levels outside of the normal range should prompt a thorough evaluation of the person's thyroid state, including the patient's T4 level, TSH level, thyroglobulin level, and anti-thyroid antibody testing.

Increased Value May Indicate: Increased T3 or free T3 levels should indicate that there is probably hyperthyroidism in the patient, particularly if the free T3 is elevated. A free T3 alone doesn't completely evaluate the thyroid gland dysfunction so other testing should be done to further evaluate the elevated T3 state. High T3 levels can be from a hyperfunction of the thyroid gland or from hyperstimulation of the T3 level from an adenoma secreting TSH in the pituitary gland. If a patient is taking anti-thyroid medications for Graves' disease, the free T3 level can be a good measurement of the patient's thyroid functioning.

Decreased Value May Indicate: Low T3 levels usually indicate a hypothyroid state. The low thyroid state can be from a low output of TSH in the pituitary gland or from hypofunction of the thyroid gland from iodine deficiency or, most likely, from Hashimoto thyroiditis, an autoimmune disease of the thyroid gland.

Factors, Risks, or Other Information: Generally, thyroid function testing and the T3 level should not be done in a patient who is ill or in the hospital because an acute illness can throw off the free T3 level and other thyroid function studies. Things that can affect the total T3 level include pregnancy, the taking of estrogen, liver dysfunction, acute illness, and resistance to thyroid hormones. Many of these things affect the total T3 level because it affects the protein levels in the body but don't affect the free T3 level, which is unaffected by protein levels. The taking of the T3 level by venipuncture is considered a relatively safe procedure.

Thyroglobulin

Abbreviation: TGB or TG

How Is It Measured: The thyroglobulin level is a serum test that is drawn from a venipuncture done on a peripheral vein, and is used from blood placed in a red top tube, a red/gold top tube, or a gold top tube from which serum is collected after centrifuging whole blood to separate the serum from the blood products. The serum thyroglobulin is then electronically determined.

Description: The thyroglobulin test is mainly used as a tumor marker that can measure the effectiveness of treatment for various kinds of thyroid cancer. Some thyroid cancers will produce thyroglobulin, which makes it a good way to evaluate whether or not the cancer has recurred after iodine treatments or a total thyroidectomy. Well-differentiated papillary cancer and follicular thyroid cancers are the two most common thyroid cancers that produce thyroglobulin. The thyroglobulin test should be drawn prior to thyroid cancer treatment to see if the tumor produces the protein. If it does, it will make a good tumor marker for treatment follow up and evaluation for recurrences. Graves' disease treatment can also be followed by evaluating the thyroglobulin level.

Indications: The primary indication for ordering a thyroglobulin test is before treatment for thyroid cancer. If the cancer secretes thyroglobulin, this test becomes a way of evaluating the effectiveness of cancer treatment. Patients with metastatic thyroid cancer that produces thyroglobulin will have persistently high levels of the hormone after a total thyroidectomy and may need chemotherapy to treat the metastases. The thyroglobulin level will also be elevated in Graves' disease so this test can be drawn as a way of measuring the degree of the disease and the effectiveness of anti-thyroid therapy.

Normal Range: The normal thyroglobulin level is 0-30 ng/ml.

Critical Range: There is no critical range for the thyroglobulin level but elevations beyond the baseline thyroglobulin level tested before treatment for thyroid cancer mean that the cancer has recurred and the patient has not had an adequate treatment for their cancer.

Increased Value May Indicate: Everyone has a low level of thyroglobulin in their body but elevations beyond 30 ng/ml may indicate Graves' disease or thyroid cancer. It is a test that is not used for the diagnosis of these diseases but is effective in monitoring the treatment of these diseases as a good tumor marker. After a total thyroidectomy or radioactive iodine treatments, the thyroglobulin level should be undetectable. Any rises after this indicate cancer recurrence and should indicate the need to search for metastases.

Decreased Value May Indicate: There are no disorders or problems associated with a low thyroglobulin level and most healthy people will have low or undetectable thyroglobulin levels.

Factors, Risks, or Other Information: High levels of thyroglobulin are not diagnostic of thyroid cancer so this can't be used as an evaluation for the disorder. A biopsy needs to be obtained to confirm the diagnosis and thyroid function testing should be done to further evaluate the possibility that the elevated thyroglobulin level is due to Graves' disease and not cancer of the thyroid gland.

4.12 Urinalysis Testing

The panel of lab values consists of:

- Dipstick Urinalysis

- Microscopic Urinalysis

Dipstick Urinalysis

Abbreviation: UA Dipstick

How Is It Measured: A dipstick urinalysis is collected from the patient after having the patient wash the urethral opening with an antiseptic and then having them void into a sterile cup. A midstream urinalysis should be evaluated as the first few milliliters of fluid can be artificially contaminated with skin bacteria and a midstream urine sample provides the most accurate diagnosis of urine abnormalities.

Description: The dipstick urinalysis is actually a set of tests on a dipstick that can evaluate the individual's urine for a variety of systemic and urinary disorders. Bladder infections, kidney problems, liver disease, and diabetes are just a few diseases that can be screened for in a dipstick urinalysis. In a dipstick urine sample, chemical testing is done on a small pad of paper placed on a dipstick. All of the pads of paper are dipped into the urine at once but it takes a differing amount of time before the test results become positive. It usually detects problems that need further evaluation and none of the dipstick tests are confirmatory of any disease.

Indications: A dipstick urinalysis is mainly done on asymptomatic patients as part of a wellness checkup or upon admission to the hospital to assess for any abnormalities. The UA dipstick will also be performed on an individual who has signs or symptoms of a urinary tract infection, such as urinary frequency, dysuria, pelvic pain, back pain, abdominal pain, polyuria, or cloudy/bloody urine.

Normal Range: There are a variety of tests done on a dipstick. In a normal urine dipstick, the urine color should be clear and yellow, the urine dipstick for glucose should be negative, the bilirubin should be negative, the ketones should be negative, the specific gravity should be between 1.003 and 1.035, the blood should be negative, the pH should be between 5.0 and 8.0, the protein should be negative, the urobilinogen should be between 0.1 and 1.0 mg/dL, the nitrate should be negative, and the leukocyte esterase should be negative.

Critical Range: There is no critical range for a dipstick urinalysis. The dipstick abnormalities seen require further workup and there are no severely dangerous results on a urine dipstick. Any abnormality found can be easily confirmed with a urine microscopic evaluation or a blood test to evaluate the blood level of the abnormal test, such as the urobilinogen level or the glucose level.

Increased Value May Indicate: The urinalysis can be interpreted in many ways. Any abnormality on the dipstick might or might not signify an internal problem so a blood workup should follow any abnormal urine dipstick. Some things that might be done if the dipstick is abnormal include a comprehensive metabolic panel, kidney studies, liver studies, a complete blood count, or a urine culture. In general, the stronger the reaction on the dipstick, the greater will the blood abnormality be when this is tested.

Decreased Value May Indicate: A urine dipstick that is negative for any abnormalities and has a normal pH and specific gravity does not mean there is any abnormality in the urine or blood and no further workup is necessary.

Factors, Risks, or Other Information: It should be noted that the urine dipstick is just a screening tool that is advantageous because it is cheap and completely painless to collect. A normal urinalysis by dipstick does not rule out any major disease but a positive finding may correctly lead to an important chemical or metabolic problem and can identify the probability of a urinary tract infection or kidney abnormality.

Microscopic Urinalysis

Abbreviation: UA Micro

How Is It Measured: A microscopic analysis of the urine is done on a clean catch specimen of the urine. A dipstick urinalysis is collected from the patient after having the patient wash the urethral opening with an antiseptic and then having them void into a sterile cup. A midstream urinalysis should be evaluated as the first few milliliters of fluid can be artificially contaminated with skin bacteria and a midstream urine sample provides the most accurate diagnosis of urine abnormalities. If there are certain abnormalities on the dipstick, such as a positive blood test, a positive leukocyte esterase test, or a positive nitrate test, a microscopic evaluation of the urine is warranted. The urine is concentrated with a centrifuge and all but about 2-4 milliliters of urine in the centrifuged urine is discarded. The bottom few milliliters are sampled with a pipette and a drop of concentrated urine is placed on the slide. A coverslip is placed over the wet mount and evaluated under the microscope.

Description: A microscopic urinalysis of a clean catch urine sample can be diagnostic of a urinary tract infection, including a kidney infection or bladder infection. The urine is collected when there is clinical evidence of a urinary tract infection, such as flank pain, pelvic pain, dysuria, hematuria, and polyuria. After a dipstick, the microscopic evaluation is performed by a trained technician.

Indications: The main indications for a urine microscopy evaluation include having symptoms of a bladder or kidney infection, or having a urine dipstick that is positive for blood, leukocyte esterase, or nitrates.

Normal Range: The microscopic urinalysis will often show several epithelial cells per high power field as the clean catch specimen is usually not perfect unless it is obtained by means of catheterization. Normal findings include a complete lack of RBCs per high power field, a complete lack of WBCs per high power field, a few epithelial cells, 0-1+ bacteria, and no urinary casts.

Critical Range: There is no critical range for a urinary microscopic evaluation. Abnormal findings usually indicate kidney disease or a urinary tract infection that can be followed up with a urine culture or an empiric treatment with antibiotics.

Increased Value May Indicate: High levels of RBCs may mean a severe bladder infection causing bleeding of the inside of the bladder or a kidney disease that causes shedding of RBCs from the renal tissue. A positive finding of bacteria and WBCs indicates a bladder infection, while the finding of RBC or WBC casts indicate abnormalities of the kidneys, including kidney diseases or a kidney infection.

Decreased Value May Indicate: Negative findings on a urine microscopic evaluation are normal and indicate no evidence of a urinary tract infection. A negative urine microscopic evaluation, however, does not rule out kidney dysfunction but usually rules out a kidney infection.

Factors, Risks, or Other Information: There are several factors that can interfere with an accurate urine microscopic evaluation. The patient needs to have a clean-catch, midstream urine for the best results. If there is an absolute need for a urine culture and accurate microscopic evaluation, catheterization may be necessary.

4.13 Stool Analysis

The panel of lab values consists of:

- Stool Evaluation for Ova Parasites
- Stool Culture

Stool Evaluation for Ova and Parasites

Abbreviation: Stool for O and P

How Is It Measured: Stool is collected usually at the time a bowel movement occurs but small amounts of stool can be obtained from a digital rectal examination. The end result should be a sample of stool in a clean, dry, covered container. In collecting a large sample, have the patient urinate first and place a plastic catch container in the toilet to catch the stool. When the stool is collected, use a clean spatula to put a walnut-sized sample of stool or about thirty milliliters of liquid stool in the container. Label the container and place it in a plastic bag.

Description: The ova and parasite or O and P evaluation is used to detect parasites in a stool sample when a parasitic infection is suspected. The ova and parasite evaluation is just one part of the total stool evaluation, which could include a stool culture for pathogenic bacteria and possibly blood tests to evaluate for the possibility of a significant gastrointestinal infection. The stool test can be checked for bacteria, parasites, and viruses at the same time. The parasitic evaluation is a microscopic evaluation of the stool for evidence of parasites or their eggs, both of which can be diagnostic of a parasitic infection of the GI tract. Other parasitic tests for stool testing include a Giardia antigen test, a Cryptosporidium antigen test, or an Entamoeba histolytica antigen test, which are blood tests that can confirm the diagnosis even if the ova and parasite evaluation is negative.

Indications: The main indications for an ova and parasite evaluation of the stool include having clinical evidence of a gastrointestinal infection, such as prolonged diarrheal symptoms, crampy abdominal pain, nausea/vomiting, and mucus or blood in the stool. People with a healthy immune system will clear the infection without any further evaluation or further treatment. Only patients who have severe dehydration, electrolyte imbalances, or other complications of GI disease need an O & P evaluation. People who have traveled to countries outside the US may also need a microscopic stool evaluation as may people who have had stream or lake water to drink.

Normal Range: A normal test would be the absence of ova and parasites in a microscopic evaluation.

Critical Range: There is no critical range for an O & P evaluation of the stool. Any findings warrant further evaluation and possible treatment.

Increased Value May Indicate: If a parasite is identified, the patient has a parasitic stool infection. The stool is evaluated for the number of ova and parasites and the parasite is identified if at all possible. The main parasites seen in the US include Giardia species from infected water, Cryptosporidium species, from infected water, and Entamoeba histolytica, which rarely is symptomatic. Worms, such as hookworms, roundworms, tapeworms, and flatworms can be identified in this type of evaluation.

Decreased Value May Indicate: The absence of ova and parasites in a stool sample does not rule out a parasitic infection and antigen levels in the blood may be necessary. A bacterium can be causing the infection so a stool sample may be warranted.

Factors, Risks, or Other Information: Most patients with Giardia, Entamoeba histolytica, and Cryptosporidium infections can have drug therapy but most resolve spontaneously within a few weeks. Patients with a healthy immune system do not have to be treated but those with an organ transplant, severe symptoms, or HIV disease usually need some kind of treatment.

Stool Culture

Abbreviation: SC

How Is It Measured: Stool is collected usually at the time a bowel movement occurs but small amounts of stool can be obtained from a digital rectal examination. The end result should be a sample of stool in a clean, dry, covered container. In collecting a large sample, have the patient urinate first and place a plastic catch container in the toilet to catch the stool. When the stool is collected, use a clean spatula to put a walnut-sized sample of stool or about thirty milliliters of liquid stool in the container. Label the container and place it in a plastic bag.

Description: A stool culture is ordered to detect the presence of pathogenic bacteria in the stool indicative of a gastrointestinal infection with any one of several pathogenic bacteria. Stool cultures can be done along with ova and parasite evaluations, GI pathogen panels, or antigen testing to completely identify the pathogen. Viruses can also be tested for in stool samples using viral analysis testing. It should be remembered that, even if a bacterial pathogen is cultured out, only a few of these infections actually need treatment as many resolve on their own. The main disease-causing bacteria include Campylobacter species, Shigella species, and Salmonella species. There are some GI pathogens that are symptomatic because of toxin production. The tests for these aren't best done by doing a culture but are better tested by checking for the toxins. Examples of these are E. coli infections and Clostridium difficile infections.

Indications: A stool culture is ordered when patients have typical signs and symptoms of a GI infection, including diarrhea, abdominal pain, fever, nausea, and vomiting. Not everyone with classical bacterial symptoms will need to have stool cultures because the infections are self-limited. Culturing of the stool can be done when there is evidence of an epidemiological outbreak of a particular species of bacteria or if the patient has severe symptoms or a poor immune system, necessitating treatment.

Normal Range: The normal range for this test is a negative culture for pathogenic bacteria.

Critical Range: There are no specific critical ranges for stool cultures. Positive cultures do not necessarily need treatment as most bacterial gastroenteritis cases are self-limited and resolve without treatment.

Increased Value May Indicate: A positive stool culture means the individual is infected with a pathogenic gastrointestinal bacterium. The most commonly positive pathogenic bacterial cultures will involve Campylobacter (found in unpasteurized milk or raw poultry), Salmonella (found in raw eggs), and Shigella (found in various kinds of contaminated food and water).

Decreased Value May Indicate: The absence of a positive stool culture may or may not indicate the presence of a bacterial gastroenteritis. Patients who are very ill and are suspected of having bacterial gastroenteritis should be treated empirically, even if the culture is negative.

Factors, Risks, or Other Information: Severe pathogenic infections of the GI tract that cause systemic complications should be treated with antibiotics; however, most patients will resolve their infections without intervention. The spread of infection should be avoided with proper hygiene and patients who are dehydrated should be instructed in oral rehydration therapy. If the infection is of an epidemiological concern, cultures may be done on selected individuals and the proper authorities should be contacted. This will help detect outbreaks that may be of local or national concern.

Chapter 5: Top 20 NCLEX Lab Values & Bonus Case Studies

Before we dive into each case study it's important to take note of the Top 20 NCLEX Lab Values and make sure you have a clear understanding of these:

1. pH
2. PaO2
3. PaCO2
4. SaO2
5. HCO3-
6. BUN
7. Total Cholesterol
8. Glucose
9. Hematocrit
10. Hemoglobin
11. HgbA1c
12. Platelets
13. Potassium
14. Sodium
15. WBC
16. Creatinine
17. Protime (PT)
18. Partial Thromboplastin Time (PTT)
19. Activated Partial Thromboplastin Time (APTT)
20. International Normalized Ratio (INR)

Case 1: pH

Patient Name: Cynthia Adams

Patient Age: 17 years

History: The patient is a junior in high school who says she just broke up with her boyfriend and admits to being distraught. She was at home talking on the phone when she developed tingling of her face, particularly around her mouth and stiffness of her fingers. Now her fingers are so stiff that both of her hands are in spasm and she says she feels extremely nervous about the sudden onset of these symptoms. Her vitals are done showing a respiratory rate of 30 and a pulse of 120. She is normotensive and appears anxious. She shows no evidence of cyanosis. An arterial blood gas is drawn.

Lab Test: pH of Arterial Blood Gas

Lab Value: pH of 7.52

Normal Range: The normal range for the arterial blood pH is 7.34 to 7.45.

Explanation: The patient is suffering from alkalosis with a pH that is above the normal range. The two main choices in any case of alkalosis is whether the alkalosis is primarily respiratory or primarily metabolic. Along with her elevated pH value, her O2 saturation is 100 percent and her arterial bicarbonate level is normal. Most likely her arterial CO2 is low, indicating that she is blowing off CO2 because of hyperventilation and anxiety. This would cause a sudden elevation of her arterial pH above the normal range from respiratory alkalosis, which is, in turn, secondary to anxiety. Her arterial bicarbonate level would be normal because the situation is acute and her kidneys would not have had the time to compensate for her elevated respiratory rate and low CO2 level.

Case 2: PaO2

Patient Name: Franklin Burns

Patient Age: 64 years

History: The patient is an older gentleman who is semi-retired. He admits to smoking 2 packs a day of mentholated cigarettes per day for the last 40 years. He is barrel-chested and admits to being short of breath at rest and says he's been like this for the last several weeks but that tonight, his shortness of breath is worse. His vital signs show a respiratory rate of 35 and a pulse of 110. His O2 saturation level is 88 percent on room air. He is slightly cyanotic around the lips and in his fingers. He has clubbing of his fingers and is leaning over a tray table as he breathes. An arterial blood gas on room air is drawn.

Lab Test: PaO2 of the arterial blood

Lab Value: PaO2 of 73 mm Hg on room air

Normal Range: The normal range for PaO2 is 80-100 mm Hg.

Explanation: The patient is cyanotic at rest and has a reduction in his arterial PaO2 is reduced, indicating he has a low partial pressure of oxygen. By history, he likely has chronic obstructive pulmonary disease and is approaching respiratory failure as would be shown to be the case if he has an elevated PaCO2 level, showing an inability to oxygenate himself on his own. Interestingly, patients with COPD have a respiratory drive to breathe that is based on their PaO2 level and their oxygen saturation level. Providing this man with oxygen based on his low PaO2 level would actually reduce his drive to breathe and would worsen his impending respiratory failure. He is likely nearing a point where he may need to be artificially ventilated should he have increased difficulty breathing.

Case 3: PaCO2

Patient Name: Anthony Evans

Patient Age: 72 years

History: The patient is an elderly gentleman who used to smoke two packs of cigarettes per day until last year when he was found to have a large cell carcinoma of the lung that was treated with a right lower lobe lobectomy, chemotherapy, and radiation to the right lung field. He is on oxygen at home but says he feels short of breath on 2 liters of oxygen at home. He presents to the emergency room with cyanosis on his portable oxygen machine. He is placed on 4 liters of oxygen in the emergency room. After thirty minutes, his oxygen saturation is 82 percent but he still has a respiratory rate of 35 breaths per minute and a pulse of 115 bpm. He has an arterial blood gas drawn on 4 liters of oxygen.

Lab Test: Partial pressure of CO2 on an arterial blood gas measurement

Lab Value: PaCO2 of 60 mmHg

Normal Range: The normal range for PaCO2 is 35-45 mmHg.

Explanation: This patient has an elevated PaCO2 in spite of having an increased respiratory rate and in spite of being on oxygen. The PaCO2 is best understood by also knowing the ph of the arterial blood, which, in his case, would likely be low because he is retaining CO2, which is acidic. He is probably always retaining some CO2 but is retaining more CO2 tonight, giving him an elevated PaCO2. He does not have full lung capacity and, for reasons that are not completely clear based on the above findings, he is approaching respiratory failure while breathing on his own. He is probably partially compensated because he has always had some respiratory acidosis but his respiratory acidosis is probably worse tonight, so he need urgent artificial ventilation to keep him ventilating at a reasonable oxygen level without such an elevation of his PaCO2.

Case 4: SaO2

Patient Name: Maria Martinez

Patient Age: 72 years old

History: The patient is an elderly woman who complains of chest pain and shortness of breath of about 10 hours duration. Her chest pain is substernal and radiates to her jaw. She has a pulse of 90 and a blood pressure of 90/50. Her respiratory rate is 29 rpm and she exhibits perioral cyanosis on room air. An oxygen saturation level is obtained on room air.

Lab Test: Oxygen saturation level

Lab Value: 85 percent

Normal Range: The normal range for oxygen saturation is 95-100 percent saturation of arterial blood.

Explanation: In this case, her oxygen saturation level was determined using a fingertip oxygen saturation level and she didn't have an arterial blood gas determination of her oxygen saturation. Would she to have an arterial blood gas determination, however, she would still probably have a low oxygen saturation level. Clinically, her chest pain and shortness of breath are characteristic of unstable angina or an acute myocardial infarction and, probably due to acute congestive heart failure and shock, she would likely have a chest x-ray showing pulmonary edema and a decreased ability to oxygenate due to fluid on her lungs. Treating her with oxygen and improving her cardiac function would probably improve her oxygen saturation level. She would benefit from 100 percent oxygen by mask, which would better oxygenate her lungs and her coronary arterial vessels until she can be definitively treated to maximize her heart and lung function.

Case 6: HCO3-

Patient Name: Samuel Abrahamson

Patient Age: 42 years

History: The patient is a middle-aged disabled man with a history of chronic renal insufficiency due to a long history of drug abuse. He is now sober and free of drugs, and is complaining of increased hand and leg edema over the last three days. He presents with vital signs that include a pulse of 85 bpm, a respiratory rate of 40, and a blood pressure of 160/110. He has obvious peripheral edema. Blood is drawn including an arterial blood gas measurement. Blood is also sent off to include a comprehensive metabolic panel.

Lab Test: Bicarbonate level of arterial blood

Lab Value: HCO3- level of 15 mmol/L

Normal Range: The normal arterial bicarbonate level is between 22 and 26 mmol/L.

Explanation: The patient has a low arterial bicarbonate level, is hyperventilating, and has a history of renal insufficiency that may be worsening recently as he is having increased problems with peripheral edema. The blood pH level would be a part of his arterial blood gas measurement and may be normal or may be low as he has a low bicarbonate level and bicarbonate is a base. The reason why his pH might be normal is that he is hyperventilating and blowing off arterial CO2 in an attempt to normalize his blood ph level. With a respiratory rate of 40, he would likely have a low PaCO2 level and would be overbreathing in an attempt to counteract a metabolic acidosis from an acute exacerbation of his renal failure and an increase in his renal excretion of bicarbonate. His metabolic panel might give clues as to his current renal status, which is likely worse than normal as the onset of his peripheral edema is relatively new. A full arterial blood gas analysis would show a low bicarbonate level, a low PaCO2 level, and a blood pH that would be low, indicating metabolic acidosis that was partially compensated for by his ventilatory status.

Case 7: BUN

Patient Name: Andrea Constantinople

Patient Age: 18 years

History: The patient is a Freshman in college who has been studying for her first set of midterms. She weighs 137 pounds and is 5 feet 4 inches tall. She admits to a long history of bulimia nervosa that is ongoing. Because she has been studying for midterms, she has been drinking less so she doesn't have to go to the bathroom, but admits she still goes to the bathroom after eating in order to purge. She says she purges up to six times per day but that this hasn't changed. She presents to the emergency department complaining of lightheadedness. Her vital signs are within normal limits except for a blood pressure of 100/50. A comprehensive metabolic panel is drawn.

Lab Test: Serum blood urea nitrogen or BUN level

Lab Value: BUN of serum of 35 mg/dL

Normal Range: The normal range for the serum BUN level is 6-20 mg/dL.

Explanation: The patient has a history of bulimia nervosa and has been both purging and restricting fluids. This places her at a high risk for dehydration. In her comprehensive metabolic panel, her serum BUN level is elevated. A serum creatinine level would also have been drawn as a part of this evaluation and would shed some light as to whether she was suffering from some sort of renal insufficiency or was simply dehydrated. Her clinical picture is that of dehydration, given her history and vital signs. The elevated serum BUN level is because she is hemoconcentrated and needs some sort of fluids. Given fluids, her clinical picture would improve and her BUN would likely normalize over several hours.

Case 8: Total Cholesterol

Patient Name: George Callahan

Patient Age: 34 years

History: This is a young, nonsmoking male who is worried because his 56-year-old father just died of a massive coronary event and he wants to make sure he has no risk factors for heart disease. He has no symptoms of heart disease or diabetes but says he's had yellow patches around his eyes since he was about twenty-five years of age. He has never had a checkup. He has a complete physical examination showing him to have a weight of 234 pounds and multiple yellow xanthomas around his eyes. He otherwise has a normal examination and normal vital signs. He has a total cholesterol panel done and a comprehensive metabolic panel drawn as well.

Lab Test: Lipid profile to include a total cholesterol level drawn on a fasting blood sample

Lab Value: Tchol of 463 mg/dL

Normal Range: A normal range for an adult having a total cholesterol reading on a fasting basis is less than 200 mg/dL.

Explanation: This is a young, overweight male with the only risk factors for heart disease being his weight, the presence of yellow xanthomas around his eyes, and a strong family history for early heart disease. His total cholesterol level puts him at a high risk for heart disease. An LDL and HDL cholesterol should also be part of this test and would likely show an elevated LDL cholesterol with a low HDL cholesterol level. A test called apolipoprotein B100 level should be drawn to see if he has a familial hypercholesterolemia level and he should be offered genetic testing. Even without genetic testing, his risk for a familial hypercholesterolemia problem is extremely high so he should be considered to have a high risk for heart disease based on his total cholesterol level. The treatment of choice is to use a statin drug such as simvastatin, atorvastatin, or lovastatin, with regular checkups for heart disease and cholesterol profiles. He needs a weight reduction diet, an exercise plan, and should be discouraged from ever smoking. He may need an exercise stress test before starting an exercise program as he may have some evidence of coronary artery disease, even at this early age.

Case 9: Glucose

Patient Name: Angela Loyola

Patient Age: 8 years

History: Angela is a school-age girl who presents to the hospital with confusion, abdominal pain, and vomiting. She has had a recent unintentional weight loss and her mother reports she's had an increased thirstiness and hungriness lately but has been very fatigued. She has otherwise been healthy except for an influenza-like illness a month ago that has mostly resolve except for the fatigue. She has a family history of rheumatoid arthritis in her maternal aunt and Crohn's colitis in her maternal grandmother, who is deceased. Her exam shows normal vital signs except for an elevated respiratory rate, and a child in some distress with abdominal pain and vomiting. She has diffuse abdominal tenderness but no focal findings. A CBC and complete metabolic panel done. Her O2 saturation is 97 percent on room air but, because she has a respiratory rate of 34 rpm, she has arterial blood gases drawn.

Lab Test: Serum glucose level

Lab Value: 548 mg/dL on a nonfasting basis

Normal Range: A normal fasting blood glucose level is between 70 to 99 mg/dL.

Explanation: Even though her glucose level is nonfasting, it is markedly elevated and she has clinical evidence for diabetic ketoacidosis. An arterial blood gas analysis would probably show a metabolic acidosis from excessive ketones in the blood, which are acidic. She should have a urinalysis and serum ketone level drawn, which probably would be elevated. She needs to have urgent IV access, correction normalize her blood glucose value and ketone levels. With her age, presentation, and family history of autoimmune disease, she likely has type 1 diabetes presenting as diabetic ketoacidosis. Once stabilized, she will need diabetic education to include information involving insulin regimens.

She will be discharged on insulin and followed closely as an outpatient, possibly by a pediatric endocrinologist.

Case 10: Hematocrit

Patient Name: Melinda Forester

Patient Age: 23 years old

History: The patient is a young woman who presents for her first obstetrical visit at 6 weeks' gestational age. This is her first pregnancy. Her history is completely unremarkable and her social history indicates that she is a nondrinker, nonsmoker, and does not use drugs. She is in a monogamous relationship as she got married four months ago. She admits to losing about 30 pounds just prior to the wedding and has kept the weight off with a low-calorie diet. She takes no medications. Her examination is unremarkable. Prenatal labs are drawn that include a CBC.

Lab Test: Hematocrit as part of a CBC evaluation

Lab Value: HCT of 29.8 percent

Normal Range: The normal hematocrit level in adult males is 41.5 percent to 50.4 percent, while the normal hematocrit for adult females is 36.9 percent to 44.6 percent.

Explanation: This is a newly pregnant woman who has recently lost a lot of weight. She has a risk of anemia because of being pregnant and because she has been dieting, and probably has had a low intake of iron-containing foods as part of a low-calorie diet. She would have indices drawn as part of her CBC, which, if she has iron-deficiency anemia would show a low MCHC and microcytic cells. An RDW would be high. Iron studies might be helpful to confirm her lack of total iron and would show both an elevated TIBC and low ferritin level. As part of her management, she would be placed on iron supplementation besides her prenatal vitamin. Her hematocrit and/or hemoglobin will be followed. Pregnancy often shows a low hematocrit so repeat iron studies might be helpful to confirm an improved iron level, reduced TIBC level, and increasing serum ferritin, indicating an improvement in iron stores. Her

HCT and/or HGB level will be followed throughout the pregnancy and, once she has normal iron stores, the iron supplement can be stopped and she can be continued on a prenatal vitamin that contains iron.

Case 11: Hemoglobin

Patient Name: Carl Thompson

Patient Age: 41 years

History: The patient is a middle-aged male who presents for a routine physical examination. He admits to several risk factors for heart disease including a sedentary lifestyle, a one-and-a-half pack a day smoking habit, and a family history of heart disease in a maternal uncle and maternal grandfather. He has never had a complete physical in the past. His exam shows a weight of 213 pounds and a mildly elevated blood pressure of 143/89. His examination is otherwise unremarkable. He has a comprehensive metabolic panel, lipid profile, and CBC with differential done on a fasting basis.

Lab Test: Fasting hemoglobin level

Lab Value: Hgb 17.1 g/dL

Normal Range: The normal hemoglobin range in adult men is 14-17.5 g/dL, while the normal hemoglobin range for females is 12.3 to 15.3 g/dL.

Explanation: The patient has an elevated fasting hemoglobin level of unknown etiology. Hemoglobin levels do not have to be fasting and it is possible but unlikely that his hemoglobin level is high because of dehydration. He has a positive smoking history, which might place him at risk for an elevated hemoglobin level on the basis of being a smoker. He would have indices and the rest of the CBC to guide the diagnosis. An oxygen saturation level might show a reduction, which would increase the chances that smoking alone is the cause of his elevated hemoglobin level. If this is normal, refer to the CBC to see if any other elements are elevated as would be seen in polycythemia vera. If the WBC and PLT levels are normal, he probably has polycythemia from smoking. With all of his risk factors for heart disease, his lipid profile and blood pressure should be carefully monitored and treated. He needs a weight loss diet, smoking cessation advice, and continual follow-up to reduce his risk factors for coronary artery disease.

Case 12: HgbA1c

Patient Name: Melanie Williamson

Patient Age: 45 years

History: Melanie is a middle-aged woman with a past medical history of type 2 diabetes since the age of 39 years. Type 2 diabetes runs in her family so she is familiar with its management. She has been on dietary control of her diabetes and has been following her blood sugars at home. She admits to multiple episodes of elevated fasting and nonfasting home blood sugar readings and says it's been hard to follow a low carbohydrate diet as she has to cook for a family of five, none of whom have diabetes at this time. Her weight is 199 pounds and her blood pressure is 140/90. The rest of her exam is unremarkable. A nonfasting HgbA1c is drawn as part of her routine diabetic follow-up.

Lab Test: Non-fasting HgbA1c on venous blood

Lab Value: 8.7 percent

Normal Range: For people without diabetes, the normal range for the hemoglobin A1c level is between 4% and 5.6%.

Explanation: Melanie is a known diabetic with an isolated non-fasting hemoglobin A1c that is elevated. She does not need to have her HgbA1c done on a fasting basis so this is a valid test indicating that dietary control of her diabetes is not working. In diabetics, the goal is to have a HgbA1c of less than 7 percent. Because she is above this level and because her blood pressure is elevated, this is probably time to promote a weight loss diet, begin metformin and lisinopril (or other ACE inhibitor), and to monitor her HgbA1c every 3-6 months. This level won't change much over time so it only needs to be completed every three to six months. The lifespan of RBCs is about 120 days so there is no purpose in checking a HbgA1c any close together than that.

Case 13: Platelets

Patient Name: Benjamin Anderson

Patient Age: 32 years

History: The patient is a young gentleman who presents for a routine physical examination. He says he's generally healthy but has noticed some increased left upper quadrant abdominal pain over the last month. He has a normal diet and does not smoke. His family history is positive for a pulmonary embolism in his father, who died after surgery on his peripheral vascular disease of a pulmonary embolism at the age of 66 years a couple of years ago. He doesn't smoke and runs several 5k races every year. His examination shows normal vital signs and an abdominal examination showing possible splenomegaly. A CBC, lipid profile, and comprehensive metabolic panel are drawn.

Lab Test: Platelet level on venous blood

Lab Value: Total platelet count of 750,000 cells per microliter

Normal Range: The normal range for the platelet count in adult males and females is 150,000 to 450,000 cells per microliter.

Explanation: The patients elevated platelet count is somewhat unexpected as he is otherwise healthy. The differential diagnosis of an elevated platelet count includes essential thrombocytosis, secondary polycythemia, primary myelofibrosis, and chronic myelogenous leukemia. The rest of his CBC will help to rule out leukemia and secondary polycythemia vera. With essential thrombocytosis, an additional workup should include genetic studies for JAK2 V617F, CALR, and MPL mutations, which would indicate a familial tendency toward having essential thrombocytosis. His left upper quadrant tenderness and findings are suggestive of splenomegaly. He is at risk for both bleeding and clotting complications later in life and should be counseled about this. People with essential thrombocytopenia have a risk for transformation to acute myelogenous leukemia in 0.6 to 6.5

percent of cases, so he should be followed for that potential complication as well as for clotting and bleeding complications.

Case 14: Potassium

Patient Name: Marcus Sampson

Patient Age: 52 years

History: The patient is a middle-aged male with essential hypertension who presents for a routine blood pressure follow up. He has done well on only hydrochlorothiazide for his hypertension and has been taking it for the past three years. He says he feels well and has been exercising regularly to keep his weight down. His blood pressure is 132/78 and his pulse is 70. He has a normal physical examination. A basic electrolyte panel is drawn because of his hydrochlorothiazide use.

Lab Test: Serum potassium (K+) level on venous blood

Lab Value: 2.9 mEq/L

Normal Range: The normal range for potassium is 3.5-5.1 mEq/L or mmol/L.

Explanation: This is a patient who has a low potassium level on hydrochlorothiazide for hypertension. He is asymptomatic; nevertheless, his low potassium level should be treated. The rest of his electrolyte panel is likely to be normal as his antihypertensive medication generally only affects the serum K+ level. His choices are to continue on HCTZ and add a potassium supplementation or to change his antihypertensive drug to any other antihypertensive or to a combination antihypertensive, such as lisinopril and hydrochlorothiazide, which is a combination ACE inhibitor and HCTZ, which often normalizes the K+ level as ACE inhibitors have a tendency to raise the K+ level.

Case 15: Sodium

Patient Name: Andrea Cortez

Patient Age: 72 years

History: The patient is an older woman who presents to the emergency department after an episode of gastroenteritis involving explosive diarrhea and vomiting. She recalls eating chicken that wasn't cooked all the way through about four days ago with the onset of diarrhea and vomiting the next day, which has been ongoing. She hasn't been able to keep any food down and has been able to drink only a limited amount of clear liquids. Her examination shows a blood pressure of 98/62, a pulse of 110 bpm, and a respiratory rate of 20 rpm. She has sunken eyes and tenting of the skin on the back of her forearm. Her weight is 110 pounds and she admits her normal weight is about 119 pounds. She is slightly confused as she doesn't remember the month but is clear on who she is and where she is. A comprehensive metabolic panel and CBC are obtained.

Lab Test: Nonfasting serum sodium (Na+) level on venous blood

Lab Value: 159 mEq/l

Normal Range: Most adults have a normal range of 136-145 mEq/l or mmol/L, while adults greater than 90 years of age have a normal range of 132-146 mEq/L or mmol/L.

Explanation: She has hypernatremia and likely has hyperchloremia as these often go together. The differential diagnosis for hypernatremia is euvolemic hypernatremia and hypovolemic hypernatremia. Her clinical picture strongly suggests hypovolemic hypernatremia from dehydration, which might also be evident by having an elevated hemoglobin and hematocrit. The treatment of choice is IV fluids to restore her total water volume. Giving IV water alone would be inappropriate as it would too quickly change her sodium level. D5W with half normal saline and some potassium would probably be appropriate as this would increase her fluid volume and decrease her sodium level gradually, reducing the chance of CNS changes from too rapidly adjusting her sodium level.

Case 16: WBC

Patient Name: Tiffany Williams

Patient Age: 3 years

History: Tiffany is a preschooler who presents to the clinic with a cough, nasal congestion, and mild shortness of breath and wheezing. She has had a cold for the last week and now has an increase in cough and chest congestion. Her examination shows a temperature of 101.2 degrees Fahrenheit, a normal blood pressure, a pulse of 110 bpm, and a respiratory rate of 26 rpm. She has purulent nasal congestion, a red left tympanic membrane, and rhonchi heard in her left lower lung field. A chest x-ray and CBC with differential are obtained as part of her workup.

Lab Test: Nonfasting WBC on venous blood

Lab Value: WBC of 23,500 wbc/mcL

Normal Range: The normal range for the WBC count is 4,500-11,000 white blood cells per microliter (mcL) for both adult men and adult women.

Explanation: Tiffany has clinical evidence of a bacterial infection of both her left ear, nasal passages, and lungs. Her chest x-ray would likely show an infiltrate. The vitals do not indicate sepsis or shock so her elevated WBC is likely due to her ear infection and pneumonia. As she is placed on antibiotics and oxygen, her WBC count will probably drop to normal within the next 24 to 48 hours and should be followed. Her differential was drawn, which, in her case, would probably show an elevated neutrophil count as the cause of her overall total elevation in WBC count.

Case 17: Creatinine

Patient Name: Tony Michaelson

Patient Age: 54 years

History: Tony is a middle-aged male with chronic type 2 diabetes since he was 43 years old. He is markedly overweight with a weight of 320 pounds that has not changed appreciably over the last ten years. He has been on metformin, lisinopril, and simvastatin and is followed regularly for his diabetes and mild hypertension. His exam shows morbid obesity and a blood pressure of 140/83, a respiratory rate of 16 rpm, and a pulse of 90 bpm. His obesity is the main finding on clinical examination. A comprehensive metabolic panel is drawn.

Lab Test: Serum creatinine with venous blood

Lab Value: 3.4 mg/dL

Normal Range: The normal range for serum creatinine level is between 0.9 mg/dL and 1.3 mg/dL in adult males and between 0.6 mg/dL and 1.1 mg/dL in adult females.

Explanation: This man is a middle-aged individual with several risk factors for renal insufficiency, the most common of which is diabetes, which is probably not in good control, and hypertension, which is only moderately in control. His age and creatinine level can help calculate his glomerular filtration rate or GFR. He can also have a 24-hour urine collection to measure his GFR, which is technically a superior test for renal failure in diabetic patients. He is nowhere near the range where he needs dialysis most likely but he needs much tighter control of his risk factors so that his serum creatinine can stay the same. At this point, he has no other reason for an elevated creatinine level other than chronic renal insufficiency. Both his creatinine level and GFR should be followed regularly to continually monitor his renal function. His HgbA1c and blood pressure should also be closely followed.

Case 18: Protime

Patient Name: Carlos Alvarez

Patient Age: 74 years

History: Carlos Alvarez is an elderly male who had an ischemic stroke a year ago and has been on warfarin since his stroke. He has been having routine measurements of his prothrombin time or protime at every doctor's visit, which is about every two to three months. He does not monitor his diet very carefully but takes his warfarin every morning with no change in his warfarin dose in the past six months. He currently takes warfarin 5 mg every day and has had no ischemic events since last year. His exam shows mild left-sided neglect and mild paresis of his left leg, which are stable since he went through physical rehabilitation after his CVA. He has a protime and INR drawn and calculated.

Lab Test: Protime on venous blood

Lab Value: 15.3 seconds

Normal Range: The normal range for a prothrombin time is 10.0-13.0 seconds.

Explanation: His protime is elevated as would be expected for someone on warfarin but it is not markedly elevated. While an INR is a better way to measure his warfarin dose; however, a protime alone can be used. While on warfarin for a CVA and for CVA prevention, the protime should be about 1.5 to 2.0 times above the normal range or approximately 20 seconds. It is possible he has taken in too much vitamin K in his diet, which has partially decreased the effectiveness of his warfarin that he needs an increase in his warfarin dose. Most likely, he needs to be counseled on foods high in vitamin K to avoid, such as leafy green vegetables, fermented soy, scallions, Brussels sprouts, cabbage, broccoli, fermented dairy products, prunes, cucumbers, and basil. If this isn't the problem, an adjustment in warfarin dosage is necessary.

Case 19: Partial Thromboplastin Time

Patient Name: Amelia Earlenson

Patient Age: 83 years

History: Amelia is an elderly woman who had an ischemic cerebrovascular accident (stroke) about two days ago. She presented within three hours of the onset of her symptoms and received tissue plasminogen activator (TPA) soon after her arrival to the emergency department. She had almost complete resolution of her aphasia and right-sided weakness within five hours on TPA is now on IV heparin and oral warfarin. Coagulation studies are done every 8 hours while she is on heparin in the hospital.

Lab Test: aPTT or activated PTT on venous blood

Lab Value: aPPT level of 59.3 seconds

Normal Range: The normal range for the aPTT is 28.5-37.5 seconds.

Explanation: The patient is a recent stroke victim on intravenous heparin and warfarin. The idea is to keep the aPTT while on heparin at about two times the normal range, which is exactly where this patient is. Her Protime also needs to be followed as she is on warfarin. When her Protime reaches 1.5 to 2.0 above the normal range or when her INR is about 1.5 to 2.0, her heparin can be stopped and she can continue with oral warfarin. At that point, she can be discharged.

Case 20: International Normalized Ratio (INR)

Patient Name: Marcus Thomlinson

Patient Age: 80 years

History: Marcus is an elderly gentleman who suffered a thrombotic event to his proximal femoral artery in his right leg two days ago. He underwent a percutaneous thrombectomy and has been on IV heparin and oral Plavix for the past two days. Because he is on intravenous heparin, he has an aPTT and INR evaluated every 8 hours. The test drawn is the aPTT with the laboratory performing a calculation of the international normalized ratio or INR, which is a more accurate way to measure the responsiveness to intravenous heparin. His aPTT is drawn as part of this routine and the INR is calculated.

Lab Test: INR on venous blood

Lab Value: INR of 1.9

Normal Range: The normal range for the INR is 0.9-1.1.

Explanation: The patient has an INR which is about two times the normal range. On patients on heparin, the goal is to have the INR between 1.5 and 2.0. His level is elevated above the normal range but is in the range of what is expected for a patient on heparin. He is on heparin to maintain a clot-free femoral artery for a few days after which the heparin will be stopped and he will be maintained on the anti-platelet drug, Plavix. At this point, no changes in his heparin dosage is recommended.

Chapter 6: Mnemonics for Lab Values

Top 20 NCLEX Labs:

1. pH
    - Metabolic Acidosis Causes: Diarrhea, Ketoacidosis, Tubules, Lactate, Salicylate = Delicate Kumquats Taste Like Sugar
    - Metabolic Alkalosis Causes: Aldosteronism, Loop diuretics, Alkali, Anticoagulants, Loss of fluid, Intake of bicarbonate = ALKALI
    - Metabolic Acidosis with increased anion gap: =Methanol, Uremia, Diabetic ketoacidosis, Propylene glycol, Isoniazid, Lactate, Ethylene glycol, Salicylates = MUDPILES
    - Respiratory Acidosis Causes: Asthma, Pulmonary edema, Scoliosis, Obesity, Neuromuscular disease, COPD = Apparently Pleasant Subjects Own Nasty Constitutions
    - Respiratory Alkalosis Causes: Hyperventilation, High altitude, Fever = Hobbits Hopped Frightfully

2. PO2
    - Causes of low PO2: Hypoventilation, Low inspired oxygen, Right to left shunt, Ventilation Perfusion impairment, Diffusion impairment= Harmful Lawnmowers Respond to Vigorously Provided Directions

3. PCO2
    - Causes of low PCO2: Hyperventilation, Hypoxia, Anxiety, Pregnancy, Pulmonary embolism=Happy Hobbits Advise Purple Pillows
    - Causes of high PCO2: Neuromuscular disorders, Chest wall disorders, CNS depression, Airway obstruction, Emphysema= Nice Caregivers Condone Adamant Efforts

4. SaO2
    - Causes of low Sa02: Hypoventilation, Low inspired oxygen, Right to left shunt, Ventilation perfusion impairment, Diffusion impairment=Hard Languages Require Verbal Discipline

5. HCO3-
    - Causes of low HCO3-: Renal failure, Diarrhea, Starvation, Diabetic ketoacidosis, Chlorthiazide use=Risky Dieticians Suggest Dutch Cuisine
    - Causes of high HCO3-: COPD, Aldosteronism, Diuretics, Severe vomiting=Certain Actions Doubt Success

6. BUN
    - BUN elevation: Azotemia, Bleeding, Catabolism, Diet (parenteral nutrition) =ABCD
    - BUN decrease: Malnutrition, Overhydration, Liver failure = Man Of Luxury

7. Cholesterol (total)
    - Causes of high cholesterol: Diet, Diabetes, Obesity, Genetics, Smoking, Sedentary lifestyle=Dead Disgusting Ghosts Organize Scary Stalkings

8. Glucose
    - Causes of high glucose: Carbohydrate intake, Diabetes, Illness, Corticosteroids, Stress, = Crimson Dots Imply Colorful Socks
    - Causes of low glucose: Physical activity, Addison's disease, Insulin, Hepatitis= Predatory Animals Increase Harm

9. Hematocrit
    - Causes of high hematocrit: Polycythemia vera, Dehydration, Lung disease, Congenital heart disease, High altitudes, Smoking =Pungent Decadent Lemons Cause Heavenly Smells
    - Causes of low hematocrit: Blood loss, Nutritional deficiencies, Aplastic Anemia, Inflammatory disease, Erythropoietin deficiency (Kidney Failure) =Building Nuts Are Industrious Engineers

10. Hemoglobin
    - Causes of high hemoglobin: Polycythemia vera, Dehydration, Lung disease, Congenital heart disease, High Altitudes, Smoking = Pretty Dainty Ladies Create Highly Amiable Situations
    - Causes of low hemoglobin: Blood loss, Nutritional deficiencies, Aplastic Anemia, Inflammatory disease, Erythropoietin deficiency (Kidney Failure) =Bright Nightlights Allow Increased Effervescence

11. Glycosylated Hemoglobin (HgbA1C)
    - Causes of high HgbA1C: Diabetes, Corticosteroids, Anemia, Genetics = Dangerous Cowboys Allow Guns

12. Platelets
    - Causes of thrombophilia: Essential thrombocytosis, Reactive thrombocytosis, Epinephrine = Efforts Require Eagerness
    - Causes of thrombocytopenia: Bone marrow suppression, Splenomegaly, Pregnancy, Infection, Hemolytic uremic syndrome, Heparin = Badly Sick Patients Inhabit Horrible Hospitals

13. Potassium
    - Causes of high potassium: Spurious causes, Kidney failure, ACE inhibitors, Burns, Addison's disease, ARBs, Rhabdomyolysis, Diabetes type I = Supportive Kind Boyfriends Are Always Really Dependable
    - Causes of low potassium: Diuretics, Diabetic ketoacidosis, Aldosteronism, Laxatives, Sweating = Dangerous Dogs Attack Lower Species

14. Sodium
    - Causes of high sodium: Dehydration, Hyperventilation, Aldosteronism, Drugs, Salt intake = Dull Humans Are Difficult Subjects
    - Causes of low sodium: Diarrhea, Cirrhosis, Kidney failure, Polydipsia, Heart failure, Diuretics, Severe vomiting = Direct Caring Knowledgeable Professors Handle Difficult Subjects

15. WBC
    - Causes of leukocytosis: Infections, Exercise, Leukemia, Bone tumors, Epinephrine, Stress = Interesting Educators Bring Easy Subjects
    - Causes of leukopenia: Viral infections, Chemotherapy, Autoimmune disease, Radiation, Splenic enlargement = Vacant Chairs Are Really Serviceable

16. Creatinine
    - Causes of high creatinine: Kidney failure, Gout, Burns, Exercise = Kinky Girls Bring Excitement
    - Causes of low creatinine: Pregnancy, Muscle mass deficiency, Aging, Liver disease, Dietary deficiency= Pink Mornings Are Lovely Dawns

17. PT
    - Causes of high protime: Vitamin K deficiency, Coumadin, Clotting Factor deficiency= Kind Caring Cute Families

18. PTT
    - Causes of high PTT: Heparin, Clotting factor deficiency=Hearty Casserole

19. APTT
    - Causes of high APTT: Heparin, Clotting factor deficiency=Hearty Casserole

20. INR
    - Causes of high INR: Vitamin K deficiency, Coumadin, Clotting Factor deficiency=Kind Caring Cute Families

Additional Important Values to Remember:

1. Chloride (Cl-)
    - Increased Chloride causes: Dehydration, Hyperventilation, Kidney disease, Cushing's disease = Dehydrated Humans Knead Cushing
    - Decreased Chloride causes: Vomiting, Gastric suctioning, CHF, Addison's disease, Metabolic alkalosis = Very Good Chlorides Are Missing

2. Magnesium (Mg+)
   - Increased Magnesium causes: Hypoparathyroidism, Kidney failure, Dehydration, Laxative abuse = Hungry Kids Dehydrate Likely
   - Decreased Magnesium causes: Malnutrition, Diabetes, Crohn's disease, Eclampsia, Burns, Hypoparathyroidism = Magnesium Deficiency Can Equal Bad Hypoparathyroidism

3. Phosphorus (PO4-)
   - Increased Phosphorus causes: High parathyroid function, Liver disease, Kidney failure, Diabetic ketoacidosis = Hurtful Levels Kill Diabetics
   - Decreased Phosphorus causes: Low parathyroid function, Diuretic abuse, Malnutrition, Antacid abuse, Diabetic ketoacidosis, Burns, Rickets = Lions Develop Malnutrition And Develop Rickets

4. Calcium (Ca+)
   - Increased Calcium causes: High Parathyroid levels, Bone cancer = Hospitals Perform Biopsies
   - Decreased Calcium causes: Spurious, Low Parathyroid levels, Alcoholism, Kidney failure, Pancreatitis = Seriously Lively Parakeets Are Keeping Pace

5. Albumin
   - Increased Albumin causes: Dehydration
   - Decreased Albumin causes: Volume expansion, Liver disease, Burns, Surgery, Low Thyroid, Diabetes, Cancer = Very Little Boys See Less Than Clearly Difficult Children

6. Basophils
   - Increased Basophil causes: Viruses, Lymphoma, Bone marrow disorders, Splenectomy, Allergies = Vacant Looks Become Super Annoying
   - Decreased Basophil causes: Allergies, Pregnancy, High Thyroid, Corticosteroid use = Angry Personalities Harm Tender Children

7. Eosinophils
   - Increased Eosinophil causes: Skin diseases, Collagen vascular disease, Allergies, Cancer, Parasites = Spirited Children Are Charming People
   - Decreased Eosinophil causes: Bone Marrow Failure = Baseball Makes Fans

8. Monocytes
   - Increased Monocyte causes: Mono, Leukemia, Inflammation, Tuberculosis = Maximal Learning Involves Teamwork
   - Decreased Monocyte causes: Bone Marrow Failure = Baseball Makes Fans

9. Neutrophils
   - Increased Neutrophil causes: Burns, Infections, Myocardial Infarction, Leukemia = Beautiful Individuals Make Interesting Partners
   - Decreased Neutrophil causes: Leukemia, HIV, Chemotherapy = Livers Harbor Cells

10. Lymphocytes
    - Increased Lymphocyte causes: Viruses, Whooping cause, Leukemia, Smoking = Virtuous Women Lack Spunk
    - Decreased Lymphocyte causes: HIV, Bone marrow failure, Common cold = Hemoglobin Benefits Children

11. Reticulocyte count
    - Increased Reticulocyte count causes: Anemia, Erythropoiesis = Analyze Equations
    - Decreased Reticulocyte causes: Bone Marrow Failure, Hemolytic anemia = Baseball Makes Families Happy

12. RBC
    - Increased RBC causes: Dehydration, Hypoxia, Erythropoietin, Polycythemia vera = Delightful Humans Exude Pizazz
    - Decreased RBC causes: Hemorrhage, Kidney failure, Anemia, Bone marrow failure = Hungry Kids Ate Better

13. MCH
    - Increased MCH causes: Large RBCs = Large Reaction
    - Decreased MCH causes: Small RBCs = Small Reaction

14. MCHC
    - Increased MCHC causes: Autoimmune Hemolytic Anemia, Burns, Spherocytosis = Attentive Humans Are Bright Students
    - Decreased MCHC causes: Iron deficiency, Thalassemia = Income Taxes

15. MCV
    - Increased MCV causes: B12 deficiency, Folate deficiency, Low Thyroid, Liver disease, Myelodysplasia = Beautiful Females Lead To Lasting Marriages
    - Decreased MCV causes: Iron deficiency, Thalassemia = Income Taxes

16. LDL Cholesterol
    - Increased LDL causes: Familial Hypercholesterolemia = Furuncles Hurt
    - Decreased LDL causes: Lipoprotein deficiency, Cirrhosis, Inflammation, High Thyroid = Leading Committees Involve Human Teamwork

17. HDL Cholesterol
    - Increased HDL causes: Healthy Level, Exercise = Healthy Lively Environment
    - Decreased HDL causes: Familial causes, Sedentary level = Fiction Sells

18. Triglycerides
    - Increased triglyceride causes: Pancreatitis, Heart Disease, = Pain Hurts Dancers

19. Rheumatoid Factor
    - Increased Rheumatoid factor causes: Rheumatoid Arthritis = Received Articles

20. Antinuclear Antibody or ANA
    - Increased ANA causes: Lupus, Autoimmune diseases = Losing Autonomy

21. Direct Coomb's test
    - Positive Direct Coomb's causes: RBC Antibodies = Reacts Acutely

22. Indirect Coomb's test
    - Positive Indirect Coomb's causes: No Transfusion = Notorious Trouble

23. Thyroid peroxidase antibody test
    - Positive thyroid peroxidase antibody test causes: Grave's disease, Hashimoto's Thyroiditis = Geriatrists Hate Tablets

24. Thyroglobulin Antibody test
    - Positive Thyroglobulin Antibody Test causes: Hashimoto's Thyroiditis, Cancer of the thyroid = Hospitals Treat Children

25. Thyroid stimulating hormone receptor antibody
    - Positive TSH receptor antibody causes: Grave's Disease = Gemstone Diamonds

26. HIV test
    - Positive HIV test is from: HIV = Hormones Improve Vitality

27. Serum iron
    - High serum iron causes: Hemochromatosis, Iron ingestion, Hemolytic Anemia, = Horrible Ideas Hurt Americans
    - Low serum iron causes: Chronic disease, Iron-deficiency Anemia = Central Intelligence Agency

28. TIBC
    - High TIBC causes: Iron-deficiency Anemia = Internal Affairs
    - Low TIBC causes: Hemochromatosis, Nephrotic syndrome, Inflammation, Liver disease Malnutrition = Hard Nights Involve Minutes

29. Ferritin
    - High Ferritin causes: Hemolytic Anemia, Sideroblastic Anemia, Iron overload, = Happy Singles Are Interesting
    - Low Ferritin causes: Iron-deficiency Anemia = Intelligence Agency

30. GFR
    - Low GFR causes: Chronic Kidney Failure = Clean, Kid-friendly Fun

31. AST
    - High AST causes: Hepatitis, Heart attacks, Muscle injury, Drugs = Heavy Husbands Marry Divas

32. ALT
    - High ALT causes: Hepatitis, Cirrhosis, Heart muscle damage, Muscle injury, Liver cancer = Harsh Customers Hate Massive Lines

33. Total Bilirubin
    - High Total Bilirubin causes: Hemolytic Anemia, Gilbert syndrome, Cirrhosis, Hepatitis = Healthy Activities Give Certain Health

34. Indirect Bilirubin
    - High Indirect Bilirubin causes: Neonatal Jaundice = Nimble Jugglers

35. Direct Bilirubin
    - High Direct Bilirubin causes: Hemolytic Anemia, Gilbert syndrome, Hepatitis, Cirrhosis = Harmful Additives Give Health Challenges

36. Ammonia
    - High Ammonia causes: Reye's syndrome, Hepatic Encephalopathy = Requirements Have Exceptions

37. TSH
    - High TSH causes: High Thyroid, Pituitary Adenoma = Hollow Trees Protect Acorns
    - Low TSH causes: Low Thyroid, Pituitary Insufficiency = Low Taxes Protect Investments

38. T4
    - High T4 causes: High Thyroid = Hamster Turds
    - Low T4 causes: Low Thyroid = Lemur Turds

39. Free T3
    - High Free T3 causes: High Thyroid = Hamster Turds
    - Low Free T3 causes: Low Thyroid = Lemur Turds

40. Thyroglobulin
    - High thyroglobulin causes: Grave's disease, Thyroid Cancer =Governments Trouble Constituents

Summary

Laboratory values reach many healthcare professionals, from the nurses and phlebotomists who gather the specimens, to the laboratory technicians, to the nurses or ward secretaries who receive the completed blood tests, and finally to the doctor who interprets the test and makes recommendations.

It is crucial to know how to properly collect a particular specimen and, for venous samples, how to collect the samples in the correct order and using the correct colored tube. Arterial specimens need to be kept on ice and need to be urgently tested. Specimens from a venipuncture may need to be mixed in the tube before properly labeling all specimens. Ideally, venipuncture samples should be sent to the lab urgently as old samples do not always have the most accurate results.

Critical values for those labs that have critical ranges should be noted and the results conveyed to the primary ordering physician as soon as possible. Much of the time, critical lab values are given verbally over the phone as well as given on paper as the lab will often recognize the need for an urgent response to the lab. As the receiving nurse, these values should be urgently recognized and taken care of as prompt treatment can be life-saving.

Hopefully, you have learned something about the most common lab values you will encounter as part of your work as a nurse. Some lab tests are primarily done in a hospital setting, while others are performed on outpatients. Remember that critical values can return on either type of laboratory testing and need attending to.

Hope you enjoyed the book!

Be sure to join our FB group by visiting:

facebook.com/groups/nursingschoolstudents/

See you in the group!

- Chase Hassen

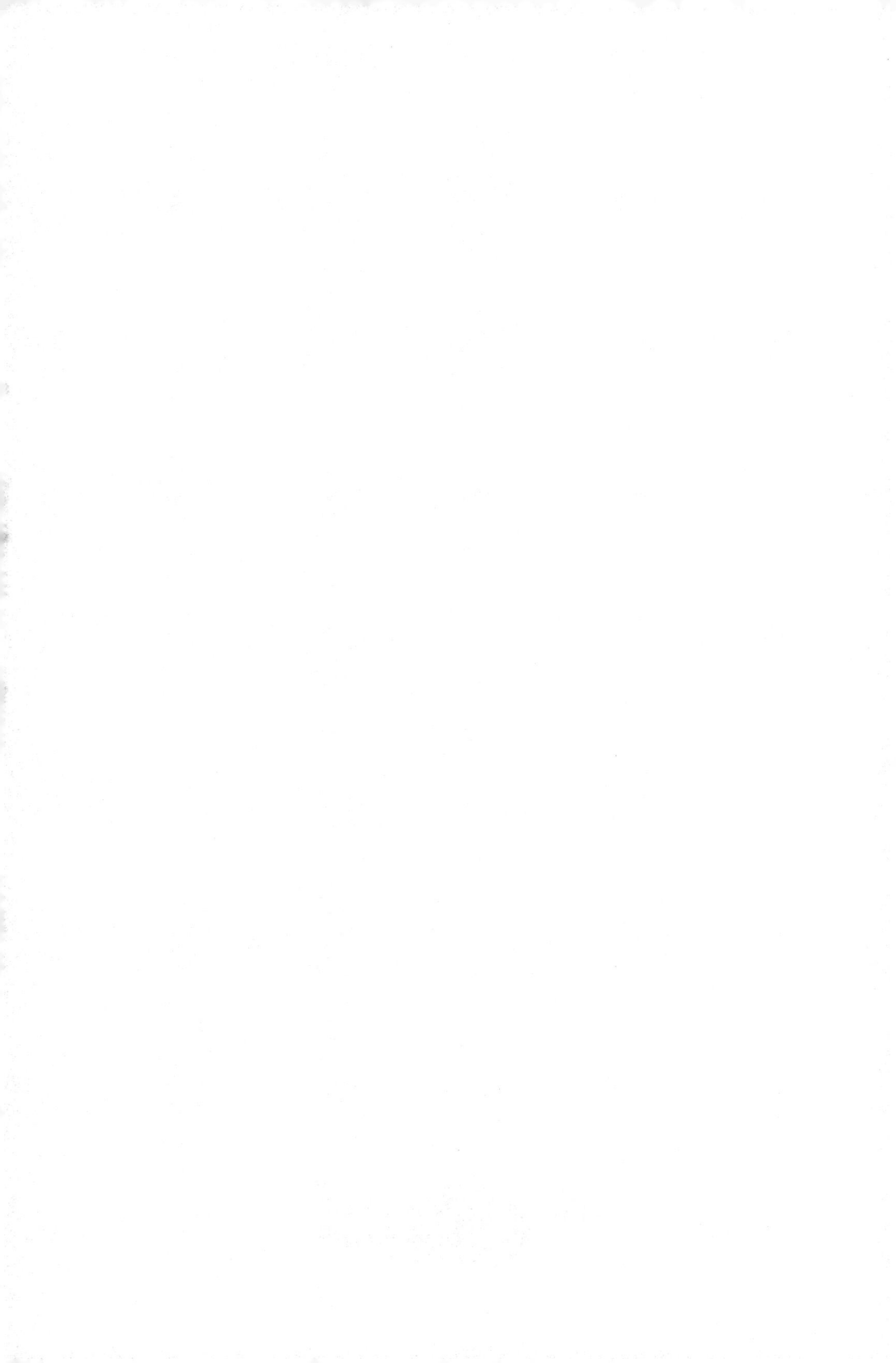

Made in the USA
Monee, IL
04 September 2022